Concepts and Definitions
of Family for the 21st Century

Concepts and Definitions of Family for the 21st Century has been co-published simultaneously as *Marriage & Family Review,* Volume 28, Numbers 3/4 1999.

The *Marriage & Family Review* Monographic "Separates"

Below is a list of "separates," which in serials librarianship means a special issue simultaneously published as a special journal issue or double-issue *and* as a "separate" hardbound monograph. (This is a format which we also call a "DocuSerial.")

"Separates" are published because specialized libraries or professionals may wish to purchase a specific thematic issue by itself in a format which can be separately cataloged and shelved, as opposed to purchasing the journal on an on-going basis. Faculty members may also more easily consider a "separate" for classroom adoption.

"Separates" are carefully classified separately with the major book jobbers so that the journal tie-in can be noted on new book order slips to avoid duplicate purchasing.

You may wish to visit Haworth's Website at . . .

http://www.haworthpressinc.com

. . . to search our online catalog for complete tables of contents of these separates and related publications.

You may also call 1-800-HAWORTH (outside US/Canada: 607-722-5857), or Fax 1-800-895-0582 (outside US/Canada: 607-771-0012), or e-mail at:

getinfo@haworthpressinc.com

Concepts and Definitions of Family for the 21st Century, edited by Barbara H. Settles, PhD, Suzanne K. Steinmetz, PhD, MSW, Gary W. Peterson, PhD, and Marvin B. Sussman, PhD (Vol. 28, No. 3/4, 1999).

The Role of the Hospitality Industry in the Lives of Individuals and Families, edited by Pamela R. Cummings, PhD, Francis A. Kwansa, PhD, and Marvin B. Sussman, PhD (Vol. 28, No. 1/2, 1998). *"A must for human resource directors and hospitality educators." (Dr. Lynn Huffman, Director, Restaurant, Hotel, and Institutional Management, Texas Tech University, Lubbock, Texas)*

Stepfamilies: History, Research, and Policy, edited by Irene Levin, PhD, and Marvin B. Sussman, PhD (Vol. 26, No. 1/2/3/4, 1997). *"A wide range of individually valuable and stimulating chapters that form a wonderfully rich menu from which readers of many different kinds will find exciting and satisfying selections." (Jon Bernardes, PhD, Principal Lecturer in Sociology, University of Wolverhampton, Castle View Dudley, United Kingdom)*

Families and Adoption, edited by Harriet E. Gross, PhD, and Marvin B. Sussman, PhD (Vol. 25, No. 1/2/3/4, 1997). *"Written in a lucid and easy-to-read style, this volume will make an invaluable contribution to the adoption literature." (Paul Sachdev, PhD, Professor, School of Social Work, Memorial University of Newfoundland, St. John's, Newfoundland, Canada)*

The Methods and Methodologies of Qualitative Family Research, edited by Jane F. Gilgun, PhD, LICSW, and Marvin B. Sussman, PhD (Vol 24, No. 1/2/3/4, 1997). *"An authoritative look at the usefulness of qualitative research methods to the family scholar." (Family Relations)*

Intercultural Variation in Family Research and Theory: Implications for Cross-National Studies, Volumes I and II, edited by Marvin B. Sussman, PhD, and Roma S. Hanks, PhD (Vol. 22, No. 1/2/3/4, and Vol. 23, No. 1/2/3/4, 1997). *Documents the development of family research in theory in societies around the world, and inspires continued cross-national collaboration on current research topics.*

Families and Law, edited by Lisa J. McIntyre, PhD, and Marvin B. Sussman, PhD (Vol. 21, No. 3/4, 1995). *With this new volume, family practitioners and scholars can begin to increase the family's position in relation to the law and legal system.*

Exemplary Social Intervention Programs for Members and Their Families, edited by David Guttmann, DSW, and Marvin B. Sussman, PhD (Vol. 21, No. 1/2, 1995). *An eye-opening look at organizations and individuals who have created model family programs that bring desired results.*

Single Parent Families: Diversity, Myths and Realities, edited by Shirley M. H. Hanson, RN, PhD, Marsha L. Heims, RN, EdD, Doris J. Julian, RN, EdD, and Marvin B. Sussman, PhD (Vol. 20, No. 12/3/4, 1994). *"Remarkable! . . . A significant work and is important reading for multidisciplinary family professionals including sociologists, educators, health care professionals, and policymakers." (Maureen Leahey, RN, PhD, Director, Outpatient Mental Health Program, Director, Family Therapy Training Program, Calgary District Hospital Group)*

Families on the Move: Immigration, Migration, and Mobility, edited by Barbara H. Settles, PhD, Daniel E. Hanks III, MS, and Marvin B. Sussman, PhD (Vol 19, No 1/2/3/4, 1993). *Examine the current research on family mobility, migration and immigration and discover new directions for understanding the relationship between mobility and family life.*

American Families and the Future: Analyses of Possible Destinies, edited by Barbara H. Settles, PhD, Roma S. Hanks, PhD, and Marvin B. Sussman, PhD (Vol. 18, No. 3/4, 1993). *This book discusses a variety of issues that face and will continue to face families in coming years and describes various strategies families can use in their decisionmaking processes.*

Publishing in Journals on the Family: Essays on Publishing, edited by Roma S. Hanks, PhD, Linda Matocha, PhD, RN, and Marvin B. Sussman, PhD (Vol. 18, No. 1/2, 1993). *This helpful book contains varied perspectives from scholars at different career stages and from editors of major publication outlets, providing readers with important information necessary to help them systemically plan a productive scholarly career.*

Publishing in Journals on the Family: A Survey and Guide for Scholars, Practitioners, and Students, edited by Roma S. Hanks, PhD, Linda Matocha, PhD, RN, and Marvin B. Sussman, PhD (Vol. 17, No. 3/4, 1992). *"Comprehensive. . . . Includes listings for some 200 social science journals whose editors have expressed an interest in publishing empirical research and theoretical articles about the family." (Reference & Research Book News)*

Wider Families: New Traditional Family Forms, edited by Teresa D. Marciano, PhD, and Marvin B. Sussman, PhD (Vol. 17, No. 1/2, 1992). *"An insightful and informative compilation of essays on the subject of wider families." (Journal of Marriage and the Family)*

Families: Intergenerational and Generational Connections, edited by Susan K. Pfeifer, PhD, and Marvin B. Sussman, PhD (Vol. 16, No. 1/2/3/4, 1991). *"The contributors challenge and move dramatically from outdated myths and stereotypes concerning who and what is family, what its members do, and how they continue its traditions to contemporary views of families and their relationships." (Contemporary Psychology)*

Corporations, Businesses, and Families, edited by Roma S. Hanks, PhD, and Marvin B. Sussman, PhD (Vol. 15, No. 3/4, 1991). *"Examines the changing relationship between family systems and work organizations." (Economic Books)*

Families in Community Settings: Interdisciplinary Perspectives, edited by Donald G. Unger, PhD, and Marvin B. Sussman, PhD (Vol. 15, No. 1/2, 1990). *"An excellent introduction in which to frame and understand the central issues." (Abraham Wandersman, PhD, Professor, Department of Psychology, University of South Carolina)*

Homosexuality and Family Relations, edited by Frederick W. Bozett, RN, DNS, and Marvin B. Sussman, PhD (Vol. 14, No. 3/4, 1990). *"Offers a smorgasbord of familial topics. . . . Provides references for those seeking more information." (Lesbian News)*

Cross-Cultural Perspectives on Families, Work, and Change, edited by Katja Boh, PhD, Giovanni Sgritta, PhD, and Marvin B. Sussman, PhD (Vol. 14, No. 1/2, 1990). *"On the cutting edge of this new perspective that sees a modern society as a set of influences that affect human beings and not just a collection of individual orphans." (John Mogey, DSc, Adjunct Professor of Sociology, Arizona State University)*

Museum Visits and Activities for Family Life Enrichment, edited by Barbara H. Butler, PhD, and Marvin B. Sussman, PhD (Vol. 13, No. 3/4, 1989). *"Very interesting reading . . . a fine synthesis of current thinking concerning families in museums." (Jane R. Glaser, Special Assistant, Office of the Assistant Secretary for Museums, Smithsonian Institution, Washington, DC)*

AIDS and Families, edited by Eleanor D. Macklin, PhD (Vol. 13, No. 1/2, 1989). *"A highly recommended book. Will provide family professionals, policymakers, and researchers with a foundation for further exploration on the largely unresearched topic of AIDS and the family." (Family Relations)*

Transitions to Parenthood, edited by Rob Palkovitz, PhD, and Marvin B. Sussman, PhD (Vol. 12, No. 3/4, 1989). *In this insightful volume, experts discuss the issues, changes, and problems involved in becoming a parent.*

Deviance and the Family, edited by Frank E. Hagan, PhD, and Marvin B. Sussman, PhD (Vol. 12, No. 1/2, 1988). *Leading experts in the fields of criminal justice, sociology, and family services explain the causes of deviance as well as the role of the family.*

Alternative Health Maintenance and Healing Systems for Families, edited by Doris Y. Wilkinson, PhD, and Marvin B. Sussman, PhD (Vol. 11, No. 3/4, 1988). *This important book offers timely discussions of current approaches and treatments in modern medicine that have had great impact upon the family health care.*

'Til Death Do Us Part: How Couples Stay Together, edited by Jeanette C. Lauer and Robert C. Lauer (Supp. #1, 1987). *"A landmark study that will serve as a classic for the emerging ethic of commitment to marriage, family, and community." (Gregory W. Brock, PhD, Professor of Family Science and Marriage and Family Therapy, University of Wisconsin)*

Childhood Disability and Family Systems, edited by Michael Ferrari, PhD, and Marvin B. Sussman, PhD (Vol. 11, No. 1/2, 1987). *A motivating book for professionals working with disabled children and their families that offers new and enlightening perspectives.*

Family Medicine: The Maturing of a Discipline, edited by William J. Doherty, PhD, Charles E. Christianson, MD, ScM, and Marvin B. Sussman, PhD (Vol. 10, No. 3/4, 1987). *"Well-written essays and a superb introduction concerning various aspects of the field of family medicine (or as it is sometimes called, family practice)." (The American Journal of Family Therapy)*

Families and the Prospect of Nuclear Attack/Holocaust, edited by Teresa D. Marciano, PhD, and Marvin B. Sussman, PhD (Vol. 10, No. 2, 1986). *Experts address the issues and effects of the continuing threat of nuclear holocaust on the behavior of families.*

The Charybdis Complex: Redemption of Rejected Marriage and Family Journal Articles, edited by Marvin B. Sussman, PhD (Vol. 10, No. 1, 1986). *An examination of the "publish-or-perish" syndrome of academic publishing, with a frank look at peer review.*

Men's Changing Roles in the Family, edited by Robert A. Lewis, PhD, and Marvin B. Sussman, PhD (Vol. 9, No. 3/4, 1986). *"Brings together a wealth of findings on men's family role enactment . . . provides a well-integrated, carefully documented summary of the literature on men's roles in the family that should be useful to both family scholars (in their own work and the classroom) and practitioners." (Contemporary Sociology)*

Families and the Energy Transition, edited by John Byrne, David A. Schulz, and Marvin B. Sussman, PhD (Vol. 9, No. 1/2, 1985). *An important appraisal of the future of energy consumption by families the the family's adaptions to decreasing energy availability.*

Pets and the Family, edited by Marvin B. Sussman, PhD (Vol. 8, No. 3/4, 1985). *"Informative and thorough coverage of what is currently known about the animal/human bond." (Canada's Mental Health)*

Personal Computers and the Family, edited by Marvin B. Sussman, PhD (Vol 8, No. 1/2, 1985). *A pioneering volume that explores the impact of the personal computer on the modern family.*

Women and the Family: Two Decades of Change, edited by Beth B. Hess, PhD, and Marvin B. Sussman, PhD (Vol. 7, No. 3/4, 1984). *"A scholarly, thorough, readable, informative,* *well-integrated, current overview of social science research on women and the family."* (*Journal of Gerontology*)

Obesity and the Family, edited by David J. Kallen, PhD, and Marvin B. Sussman, PhD (Vol. 7, No. 1/2, 1984). *"Should be required reading for all persons touched by the problem of obesity–the teachers, the practitioners of every discipline, and the obese themselves."* (*Journal of Nutrition Education*)

Human Sexuality and the Family, edited by James W. Maddock, PhD, Gerhard Neubeck, EdD, and Marvin B. Sussman, PhD (Vol. 6, No. 3/4, 1984). *"Twelve chapters that not only add some new ideas about the place of sexuality in the family but also go beyond this to show how widely sexuality influences human behavior and thought . . . excellent."* (*Siecus Report*)

Social Stress and the Family: Advances and Developments in Family Stress Theory and Research, edited by Hamilton I. McCubbin, Marvin B. Sussman, PhD, and Joan M. Patterson (Vol. 6, No. 1/2, 1983). *An informative anthology of recent theory and research developments pertinent to family stress.*

The Ties That Bind: Men's and Women's Social Networks, edited by Laura Lein, PhD, and Marvin B. Sussman, PhD (Vol. 5, No. 4, 1983). *An examination of the networks for men and women in a variety of social contexts.*

Family Systems and Inheritance Patterns, edited by Judith N. Cates and Marvin B. Sussman, PhD (Vol. 5, No. 3, 1983). *Specialists in economics, law, psychology, and sociology provide a comprehensive examination of the disposition of property following a death.*

Alternatives to Traditional Family Living, edited by Harriet Gross, PhD, and Marvin B. Sussman, PhD (Vol. 5, No. 2, 1982). *"Professionals interested in the lifestyles described will find well-written essays on these topics."* (*The Amercian Journal of Family Therapy*)

Intermarriage in the United States, edited by Gary A. Crester, PhD, and Joseph J. Leon, PhD (Vol. 5, No. 1, 1982). *"A very good compendium of knowledge and of theoretical and technical issues in the study of intermarriage."* (*Journal of Comparative Family Studies*)

Cults and the Family, edited by Florence Kaslow, PhD, and Marvin B. Sussman, PhD (Vol. 4, No. 3/4, 1982). *"Enlightens not only the professional but the lay reader as well. It provides support and understanding for families . . . gives insight and . . . enables parents, friends, and loved ones to better understand what happens when one joins a cult."* (*The Family Psychologist*)

Family Medicine: A New Approach to Health Care, edited by Betty Cogswell and Marvin B. Sussman (Vol. 4, No. 1/2, 1982). *The history, rationale, and the continuing developments in this medical specialty all in one readable volume.*

Marriage and the Family: Current Critical Issues, edited by Marvin B. Sussman (Vol. 1, No. 1, 1979). *Covers pluralistic family forms, family violence, never married persons, dual career families, the "roleless" role (widowhood), and non-marital, heterosexual cohabitation.*

Concepts and Definitions of Family for the 21st Century has been co-published simultaneously as *Marriage & Family Review*™, Volume 28, Numbers 3/4 1999.

Cover design by Thomas J. Mayshock Jr.

Library of Congress Cataloging-in-Publication Data

Concepts and definitions of family for the 21st century / Barbara H. Settles . . . [et al.] editors.
    p. cm.
    Includes bibliographical references and index.
    ISBN 0-7890-0765-7 (alk. paper)
    1. Family. I. Settles, Barbara H.
HQ518.C655 1999
306.85–dc21

99-31588
CIP

Concepts and Definitions of Family for the 21st Century

Barbara H. Settles
Suzanne K. Steinmetz
Gary W. Peterson
Marvin B. Sussman
Editors

Concepts and Definitions of Family for the 21st Century has been co-published simultaneously as *Marriage & Family Review,* Volume 28, Numbers 3/4 1999.

The Haworth Press, Inc.
New York • London • Oxford

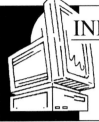

INDEXING & ABSTRACTING

Contributions to this publication are selectively indexed or abstracted in print, electronic, online, or CD-ROM version(s) of the reference tools and information services listed below. This list is current as of the copyright date of this publication. See the end of this section for additional notes.

- *Abstracts in Social Gerontology: Current Literature on Aging*
- *Abstracts of Research in Pastoral Care & Counseling*
- *Academic Abstracts/CD-ROM*
- *Academic Search: database of 2,000 selected academic serials, updated monthly*
- *AGRICOLA Database*
- *Applied Social Sciences Index & Abstracts (ASSIA) (Online: ASSI via Data-Star) (CDRom: ASSIA Plus)*
- *BUBL Information Service, an Internet-based Information Service for the UK higher education community*
- *CNPIEC Reference Guide: Chinese National Directory of Foreign Periodicals*
- *Contemporary Women's Issues*
- *Current Contents: Clinical Medicine/Life Sciences (CC:CM/LS) (weekly Table of Contents Service), and Social Science Citation Index. Articles also searchable through Social SciSearch, ISI's online database and in ISI's Research Alert current awareness service*
- *Expanded Academic Index*
- *Family Studies Database (online and CD/ROM)*
- *Family Violence & Sexual Assault Bulletin*
- *GenderWatch*
- *Guide to Social Science and Religion*
- *IBZ International Bibliography of Periodical Literature*
- *Index to Periodical Articles Related to Law*
- *MasterFILE: updated database from EBSCO Publishing*
- *PASCAL, c/o Institute de L'Information Scientifique et Technique*

(continued)

- *Periodical Abstracts, Research I (general & basic reference indexing & abstracting data-base from University Microfilms International (UMI))*
- *Periodical Abstracts, Research II (broad coverage indexing & abstracting data-base from University Microfilms International (UMI))*
- *Population Index*
- *Psychological Abstracts (PsycINFO)*
- *Sage Family Studies Abstracts (SFSA)*
- *Social Planning/Policy & Development Abstracts (SOPODA)*
- *Social Science Source: coverage of 400 journals in the social sciences area, updated monthly, EBSCO Publishing*
- *Social Sciences Index (from Volume 1 & continuing)*
- *Social Work Abstracts*
- *Sociological Abstracts (SA)*
- *Special Educational Needs Abstracts*
- *Studies on Women Abstracts*
- *Violence and Abuse Abstracts: A Review of Current Literature on Interpersonal Violence (VAA)*

Special Bibliographic Notes related to special journal issues (separates) and indexing/abstracting:

- indexing/abstracting services in this list will also cover material in any "separate" that is co-published simultaneously with Haworth's special thematic journal issue or DocuSerial. Indexing/abstracting usually covers material at the article/chapter level.
- monographic co-editions are intended for either non-subscribers or libraries which intend to purchase a second copy for their circulating collections.
- monographic co-editions are reported to all jobbers/wholesalers/approval plans. The source journal is listed as the "series" to assist the prevention of duplicate purchasing in the same manner utilized for books-in-series.
- to facilitate user/access services all indexing/abstracting services are encouraged to utilize the co-indexing entry note indicated at the bottom of the first page of each article/chapter/contribution.
- this is intended to assist a library user of any reference tool (whether print, electronic, online, or CD-ROM) to locate the monographic version if the library has purchased this version but not a subscription to the source journal.
- individual articles/chapters in any Haworth publication are also available through the Haworth Document Delivery Service (HDDS).

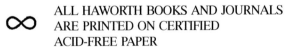

Concepts and Definitions
of Family for the 21st Century

CONTENTS

ABOUT THE EDITORS

Barbara H. Settles, PhD, is Professor of Individual and Family Studies and Senior Policy Fellow, Center for Community Development and Family Policy at the University of Delaware, Newark, Delaware, and is a well-recognized national and international scholar in the field of family studies. She received her education at The Ohio State University and the Merrill Palmer Institute. She is President of the Committee for Family Research of the International Sociological Association, Past President of Groves Conference on Marriage and Family Life and the Family Science Association, and President-elect, Delaware-Panama Partners in the Americas, and is also a life member or fellow of several major academic associations. Dr. Settles is co-editor and author of *Advanced Family Science, Families on the Move: Migration, Immigration, Emigration and Mobility,* and *American Families and the Future: Analysis of Possible Destinies.* She has also published numerous articles and chapters including major chapters on the future of families in the *Handbook of Marriage and the Family* (1st and 2nd editions).

Suzanne K. Steinmetz, PhD, MSW, DAPA, is Professor and former Chair of Sociology at Indiana University-Purdue University at Indianapolis (IUPUI). She is certified as a civil and family mediator and mediates neighborhood disputes for Indianapolis Superior Courts. Dr. Steinmetz does pro bono therapy with a focus on individuals with a diagnosis of Dissociative Identity Disorder. Credited as being one of the founders of the field of family violence, she was the first scholar to bring the problem of battered husbands and elder abuse into the public arena as a result of her congressional testimony in 1978. She served on the Board of Directors of the Society for the Study for Social Problems and was President of both the University of Delaware's and Indiana University's chapters of Sigma Xi, the National Science Society. Steinmetz has authored two research monographs, *Duty Bound: Elder Abuse and Family Care,* and *Cycle of Violence: Assertive, Aggressive and Abusive Family Interaction*; co-authored *Behind Closed Doors: Violence in American Families* and *Marriage and Family Reality: Historical and Contemporary Analysis*; and edited *Family and Support Systems Across* *the Life Span* and *Violence in the Family*. She also co-edited *Handbook of Marriage and the Family* (1st and 2nd editions) and *Sourcebook of Family Theory and Methods: A Contextual Approach*, two major reference books in the discipline. Steinmetz has also authored over 70 additional publications, and produced a curriculum for reducing conflict and violence in the school (K-9), two videos on elder abuse, and a computerized decision-making game for adolescents.

Gary W. Peterson, PhD, is Professor and Chair of the Department of Sociology at Arizona State University. He is also former Chair of the Department of Family Resources and Human Development, and has an Adjunct Faculty appointment in this department. Dr. Peterson's general area of research and scholarly expertise is adolescent development within the context of family and parent-child relationships. Currently, he is analyzing the impact of ethnic and cultural issues in samples of adolescents from the Peoples' Republic of China, Russia, India, Mexico, Chile, and the U.S. Previous research using samples from the U.S. examined health issues in Mexican-American populations of adolescents and young adults as well as influences on the life plans of low-income, rural youth from Appalachian areas of the United States. Peterson's research papers have appeared in such publications as *Journal of Marriage and the Family, Family Relations, Journal of Adolescent Research, Youth and Society, Family Science Review, Family Process,* and *Family Issues.* He was co-editor of *Handbook of Marriage and the Family* (2nd ed.) and *Adolescents in Families.* Major review articles on parent-child and parent-adolescent relationships have appeared in several books including *Advances in Adolescent Development, Handbook for Family Diversity, Handbook of Marriage and the Family* (1st and 2nd editions), and *Families Across Time: A Life Course Perspective.* Dr. Peterson has been a guest editor for special issues of several research journals and has been a member of the Board of Directors for the National Council on Family Relations.

Marvin B. Sussman, PhD, is UNIDEL Professor of Human Behavior Emeritus at the College of Human Resources, University of Delaware, and Member of the CORE Faculty, College of Interdisciplinary Arts and Sciences, Union Institute, Cincinnati, Ohio. A member of many professional organizations, he was awarded the 1980 Ernest W. Burgess Award of the National Council on Family Relations. In 1983, he was elected to the prestigious Academy of Groves for scholarly contributions to the field, as well as awarded a life-long membership for services to the Groves Conference on Marriage and the Family in 1984. Dr. Sussman received the Distinguished Family Award of the Society for the Study of Social Problems (1985) and the Lee Founders Award (1992), SSSP's highest professional award. Also in 1992 he was the recipient of the State of Delaware Gerontological Society Award for contributions to research and education in the family and aging fields. Dr. Sussman has published over 250 articles and books on family, community, rehabilitation, organizations, health and aging.

Introduction

This volume entitled *Concepts and Definitions of Family for the 21st Century* was reviewed and accepted by Professor Sussman and it is a most appropriate topic. Following World War II, scholars continued a trend first noted by Saint-Simon, Durkheim, Weber, Simmel, and Marx, sociologists who examined the impact of industrialization and modernization on society.

George Murdock's examination of countless societies throughout the world resulted in his proclamation that as societies modernized they became nuclear family–a universal form. Talcott Parson, especially, was in the forefront of contemporary scholars who saw any change in the traditional family, where father was the head and fulfilled instrumental roles and mothers served the nurturing, expressive roles, as leading to a breakdown of this universal family form. Although the romantic view of family as a multigenerational, close-knit family, residing together, has now been amply laid to rest, during the 1950s there was considerable concern that young families living in their own homes was an indicator that nuclear families were disconnecting from their kin.

Throughout his career Sussman has answered naysayers' statements regarding the downfall of the family with his research documenting precisely what was occurring. His own early work challenged that suggested by Parsons and other Structural-Functionalists regarding the desirability as well as universality of the nuclear family form. He brought attention to the strength of families across the generations in his landmark article published in *Social Problems* in 1959 entitled "The Isolated Nuclear Family: Fact or Fiction." Research, instead of ideology, was used to demonstrate that industrialization may have modified the nuclear family in appearance and residential arrangements, but kinship ties were not destroyed and the nuclear family was not isolated from kin connections. Other research conducted by Sussman focused on intergenerational support, diversity in defining family membership, and change in family structures and functions.

[Haworth co-indexing entry note]: "Introduction." Steinmetz, Suzanne K., and Gary W. Peterson. Co-published simultaneously in *Marriage & Family Review* (The Haworth Press, Inc.) Vol. 28, No. 3/4, 1999, pp. 1-2; and: *Concepts and Definitions of Family for the 21st Century* (ed: Barbara H. Settles et al.) The Haworth Press, Inc., 1999, pp. 1-2. Single or multiple copies of this article are available for a fee from The Haworth Document Delivery Service [1-800-342-9678, 9:00 a.m. - 5:00 p.m. (EST). E-mail address: getinfo@haworthpressinc.com].

The focus of this volume also documents Sussman's driving force to view family not just from a U.S. perspective, but to be inclusive in the view of family from many cultures and many societies. Not only did he conduct some of the first cross-national research on families, but he mentored (and continues to do so) countless sociologists and family scholars throughout the world. This issue contains work by scholars in Israel, Sweden, Lithuania, United Kingdom, Norway, and Canada as well as the United States.

A number of these articles were first presented as concept papers at a Committee on Family Research of the International Sociological Association organized by Jan Trost and Irene Levin. Barbara Settles took responsibility for inviting additional authors to prepare papers on this topic and provided editorial assistance; Andy Settles took responsibility for technical editing and other areas of pre-production. We were greatly assisted by the considerable preliminary work that they had provided and we wish to acknowledge and thank them for their valuable assistance.

Suzanne K. Steinmetz
Gary W. Peterson
Co-Editors-Elect, Marriage & Family Review

SECTION I:
THEORETICAL
AND HISTORICAL APPROACHES

What Is Family?
Further Thoughts
on a Social Constructionist Approach

James A. Holstein
Jay Gubrium

INTRODUCTION

The question "What is family?" is still controversial. The issue has become an increasingly important social policy concern in recent years as descriptions of traditional living arrangements and social relations don't seem to apply as they once did (Stacey, 1990; Cheal, 1993). On the academic front, the question continues to animate family studies, with scholars and

James A. Holstein is affiliated with the Department of Sociology and Cultured Sciences, Marquette University, P.O. Box 1881, Milwaukee, WI 53201-1881.

Jay Gubrium is affiliated with the Department of Sociology, University of Florida, Gainesville, FL 32611.

[Haworth co-indexing entry note]: "What Is Family? Further Thoughts on a Social Constructionist Approach." Holstein, James A., and Jay Gubrium. Co-published simultaneously in *Marriage & Family Review* (The Haworth Press, Inc.) Vol. 28, No. 3/4, 1999, pp. 3-20; and: *Concepts and Definitions of Family for the 21st Century* (ed: Barbara H. Settles et al.) The Haworth Press, Inc., 1999, pp. 3-20. Single or multiple copies of this article are available for a fee from The Haworth Document Delivery Service [1-800-342-9678, 9:00 a.m. - 5:00 p.m. (EST). E-mail address: getinfo@haworthpressinc.com].

3

researchers taking various positions on the way "family" should be defined and studied (Boss, Doherty, LaRossa, Schumm & Steinmetz, 1993; Bernardes, 1997; Levin, 1993).

As we have listened to swirling political and intellectual debates about what social arrangements should or should not be considered "family," in both theoretical and "real life" contexts, we have become increasingly interested in these exchanges in their own right. Indeed, over the years, we have come to view discussions concerning family order, membership, and meaning–in all variety of everyday situations–as most telling in determining "what is family." It's not that we think these discussions can ultimately discern the objective truth of the matter. Rather, we've come to view *family discourse* as a social process by which "family," as a social form, is brought into being as a matter of practice, so to speak. Following this observation, we've developed an analytic perspective that looks at "family" in terms of its social construction. Our aim is to empirically document the myriad social processes through which persons in the course of everyday life produce and organize "family" as a meaningful designation for social relations.

This approach is part of what some have called a paradigm shift in family studies (Allen & Demo, 1995), a trend towards more inclusive family theorizing and research (Baca Zinn, 1992) that increasingly recognizes family pluralism and diversity (Baber & Allen, 1992; Thompson, 1992; Walker, 1993). At the same time, it challenges standard ways of conceptualizing family by questioning the notion of family as a determinate social form that corresponds to any singular or monolithic concept of *the family* written large. The constructionist perspective orients to the following sorts of questions: In a world of myriad and competing interpretations of domestic life, how is family defined and experienced? Who or what defines the substance and organization of domestic life? How are the parameters of family meanings established?

This article briefly outlines our constructionist approach to family studies (Gubrium & Holstein, 1987, 1990, 1993a; Holstein & Gubrium, 1994, 1995a). First, we describe how an ethnomethodologically-informed analytic viewpoint is brought to bear on the social construction of family. In responding to the question "What is family?" we argue that family is not objectively meaningful–that it does not take on the substantive contours of a specific ideal, past or present. Instead, we maintain that it is constantly under construction, obtaining its defining characteristics somewhere, somehow, in real time and place, through interpretive practice. After discussing the theoretical underpinnings, methodological imperatives, and analytic implications of the constructionist approach, we then address some questions and concerns that have been raised about trying to describe and analyze family as a product of social construction.

ANALYZING "FAMILY" AS INTERPRETIVE PRACTICE

Taking the position that family is socially constructed leads researchers to study family as a constellation of ideas, images, or terminology that is *used* to assign meaning to aspects of everyday life (Bernardes, 1993, 1997; Gubrium & Holstein, 1987, 1990, 1993a, 1993b; Holstein & Gubrium, 1994a, 1995; Hopper, 1993; Miller, G., 1991; Miller, L., 1990a, 1990b; Rosenblatt, 1994). This means that the constructionist approach engages a topic that differs significantly from that of conventional family studies. Traditional approaches typically assume that *the* family, or even diverse family forms, exist as part of everyday reality in some objective condition, apart from acts of interpretation. Research typically attempts to describe and explain what goes on in and around the family unit. Because families are assumed to be located in households, unobtrusive access is a general concern. Naturalistic qualitative approaches in particular emphasize the inconspicuous observation of families in their natural habitat, with the goal of producing rich descriptions of family members' experience or points of view (Rosenblatt & Fischer, 1993).

The constructionist approach, in contrast, considers family to be an idea or configuration of meanings, thus problematizing its experiential reality. The objective is to understand *how* family meanings are assembled and *used* in any site or social location, and *how* this situated process of interpretation gets transmuted into concrete domestic life. In order to convey both the socially active, agentic side of family construction and the substantive resources and experiential circumstances that condition interpretation, we conceptualize the production of domestic order in terms of *interpretive practice*–the procedures, conditions, and resources through which reality is apprehended, understood, organized, and represented in the course of everyday life (Gubrium & Holstein, 1997; Holstein, 1993; Holstein & Gubrium, 1994b).

This view of family as a matter of interpretive practice is quite different from the conventional vision of family as a group or object to be described and explained. Indeed, it interpretively transforms family from a concrete collectivity into an interactional artifact of the process of interpreting social relations. "Family" and related terms of reference become an interpretive vocabulary, a set of conceptual resources for *accomplishing* the meaning of social bonds. Concretely, what comes to be known and understood as domestic order (or disorder) is constructed through family discourse, making family an interactional achievement.

The Artful Side of Interpretation

As a matter of interpretive practice, the construction of family has both its active and substantive sides. When Harold Garfinkel (1967) set out his vision for ethnomethodology, he used the term "artful" to convey how adroitly, spontaneously, resourcefully, and creatively people accomplish social order. The term refers to the myriad processes and procedures that everyday actors engage as they produce, moment-by-moment, the realities they inhabit. Most importantly, interacting persons artfully produce reality by "doing things with words," "talking reality into being," in a manner of speaking. Garfinkel's term is an apt one for characterizing the construction of families because it sensitizes us to the individual agency that is implicated in the assignment of domestic meaning.

Consider, for example, the interpretations of domestic ties and family structure that are documented in Carol Stack's now classic ethnography of an African-American community, *All Our Kin* (1974). In the following extract, Billy, a young African-American woman living in a Midwestern city, describes the family ties structuring her daily life:

> Most people kin to me are in this neighborhood . . . but I got people in the South, in Chicago, and in Ohio too. I couldn't tell most of their names and most of them aren't really kinfolk to me. . . . Take my father, he's no father to me. I ain't got but one daddy and that's Jason. The one who raised me. My kids' daddies, that's something else, all their daddies' people really take to them–they always doing things and making a fuss about them. We help each other out and that's what kinfolks are all about. (p. 4)

Here, Billy projects family structure and meaning by convincingly articulating a familiar, recognizable vocabulary with features of her day-to-day life in order to construct and convey what it means to be family. She uses a language of care and cooperation to establish the parameters of her "family." By actively assigning family status in this way, Billy indicates what persons mean to one another, simultaneously designating their interpersonal rights and obligations. She instructs her listeners in how to interpret and understand the concrete meaning of particular social ties, publicly constituting domestic order in relation to the practical circumstances that compose the life world that she confronts daily.

Compare this with the interpretations of family that we often encounter in social service agencies, courts, or political forums. Think of how often we hear family defined in a language of biological ties or legal status, in terms of the traditional unit of married parents and their offspring. This image is offered as both the moral and legal foundation of responsible society. In such instances, culturally popular terminology is invoked to define the domestic unit. For example, Dorothy Smith (1993) notes that the relatively standardized template of meanings (the ideological code of the "Standard North American Family") conveys what it means to be a family in legal, moral, and biological kinship terms. Such concepts, however, do not communicate meaning in terms of commitment, caring, and obligation that Billy employed in the above extract. Responding to a different configuration of concerns, the second definition offers a rendition of family that is equally recognizable, yet strikingly different from Billy's version.

Our aim here is not merely to suggest that persons define and describe social relations to suit their own needs. Nor is it to suggest that some family definitions are more legitimate or authentic than others. Our concerns are more epistemological. The contrasting scenarios show us that family structure and meaning are artfully executed interactional projects that are conditioned by decidedly public circumstances and practical concerns. From this perspective, the essence of family is found in the way family is *used*, not in conventional or idealized social forms.

This view of *family-in-use* intentionally evokes an active view of reality construction. This is characteristic of the ethnomethodological sensibilities that inform our perspective. While the approach derives from phenomenological initiatives (Berger & Luckmann, 1966; Schutz, 1970), the version we are presenting reflects ethnomethodology's abiding concern for the interactional bases of reality construction (Garfinkel, 1967; Heritage, 1984; Pollner, 1987). Social phenomenologists Peter Berger and Thomas Luckmann (1966) suggest that social institutions, once constructed, are virtually self-maintaining in the absence of problems or challenges; institutions "tend to persist unless they become 'problematic'" (p. 117). Ethnomethodology, in contrast, construes institutional realities as ongoing, locally-managed accomplishments. Rather than treating institutions as self-sustaining, it focuses on how constitutive actions continually produce and reproduce local realities, with context and interpretive process being reflexively related (Heritage, 1984). Thus, an ethnomethodologically-informed constructionist approach to family emphasizes interaction as mediating family meaning and domestic reality. It is more concerned with the articulation of domestic meanings than with the "finite province of meanings" that comprises family (McLain & Weigert, 1979) or the cognitive principles that sustain "the" family as a social form. Its focus is on family *usage* as a source of domestic meaning and order (Holstein, 1988).

Conditions of Interpretation

As Karl Marx (1964) reminds us, however, people do not construct their lives completely according to their own desires. While the social construction of family is artful, it is not without social bounds. Domestic order is not assembled from the ground up on each interpretive occasion. Rather, the process is mediated by the interpretive resources and circumstances at hand. Interpretation is conditioned by practical exigencies, relying on delimited cultural categories–collective representations, in Emile Durkheim's (1961) terms–that are diversely articulated with, and attached to, experience. We refer to these interpretive resources and parameters as *local culture* (Gubrium, 1989).

Culture, from this perspective, is not a set of prescriptions or rules for interpretation and action; rather, it is a constellation of more or less regularized, localized ways of assigning meaning and responding to things. It provides familiar interpretive resources and standards of accountability to which community members must orient as they formulate their actions. By characterizing culture as local, we are suggesting that it comprises the proximate, ordinary, circumstantial particulars that are taken into account and used to establish the meaningful objects and events of everyday life.

Local culture is thus a situationally assembled array of resources and conditions for interpretation, not a monolithic set of injunctions or absolute directives. Like Michel Foucault's (1973) notion of the institutional gaze, local culture may "incite" (Foucault, 1979) particular interpretations and supply the vocabulary for their articulation, but it neither dictates nor determines what is interpretively constructed.

Considering family discourse from this standpoint, local cultures of domesticity convey relatively stable and distinct ways of conceptualizing family, posing delimited conditions of interpretation that are, in turn, subject to interpretive practice. For example, a family therapy program conceiving of the family as a configuration of sentiments provides participants with a particular orientation and vocabulary for interpreting and portraying domestic troubles, to be articulated in the language of feelings and sharing. Another therapy agency, with its corresponding image of the family as a hierarchy of authority, would formulate family order and disorder quite differently, in terms of power and authority (Gubrium, 1992). It is quite possible, therefore, for staff members in one agency to discern family order in the same domestic circumstances that would be viewed as dysfunctional in another agency. While far from totalized or deterministic, local culture thus offers different ways of thinking and talking about experience, providing interpretive tools and materials that can be used to fashion meaning.

Interpretation in contemporary life is further conditioned by the diverse ways organizations invoke local culture. The structure of organizational relations–such as specialized mandates and missions, or professional and occupational outlooks and orientations–provides additional resources for constructing domestic relations. To the extent that localized configurations of domestic meaning are mediated by particular perspectives or positions in a setting, we consider the meaning-making process to be *organizationally embedded* (Gubrium, 1987).

Professional outlooks and agendas thus combine to influence the local assignment of meaning in distinctive ways. A judge in an involuntary commitment hearing, for example, would be concerned about the need to contain the

practical issues. We conclude this article by anticipating some of these concerns and taking the opportunity to address them.

Methodological Concerns

Because our approach orients to family discourse as a way of assigning meaning to relationships, it directs the researcher's attention to talk and interaction. Examining the dynamic course of social encounters, it is apparent that the meanings of social relations are not set in stone, but may be articulated in many ways. Relationships are multifaceted, extensive in scope, and enduringly subject to interpretation. To "mother" someone, for example, suggests a nurturing relationship. While the term refers to a recognizable familial role, it may or may not be applied in the context of formal familial linkages. Moreover, the context of use will affect the nuance of meaning.

From a research perspective, the question is, does this mean that systematic inquiry into the social construction of the family orients to an interpretive "free-for-all"? Does it suggest that the study of family construction is the documentation of whatever serves to define or undefine relationships as familial, whenever or wherever they occur, in or out of households, regardless of whether they are applied to conventional familial bonds?

The answer is yes, in a sense, it does. But not just *anything* goes! Methodologically, the constructionist family researcher should be prepared to go wherever talk and social interaction orients to relationships in familial terms. As we noted earlier, family interpretation is increasingly deprivatized, taking place in myriad locales beyond the household. In contemporary life, what is or is not family is defined as much in nonfamilial institutional contexts as in the privacy of the home. Accordingly, family members who have cohabited for decades, for example, may learn for the first time what they mean and, in practice, what they have been, to each other during a meeting of a multi-family support group for the parents of substance abusing adolescents. As far from home as this venue might be, it is the consequential scene for defining domestic relations. Interpretively, the familial is realized–both understood and assigned its reality–on any occasions that it is made a topic of discussion. It is only in this sense that "anything goes."

This is far from interpretive chaos. Methodologically, the constructionist researcher must also be prepared to take account of the working conditions of interpretation. While people are free, in principle, to assign or withdraw a familial designation from any relationship, there are definite practical consequences for doing so. The use of the term "mother," for example, does not occur in a definitional vacuum, but is communicated and received against the cultural and institutional contexts of the relationship to which it is applied. A reference to the chair of a university department as someone who "mothers" her (or his) faculty may turn the researcher's attention to the chair's and faculty members' interpersonal sentiments and defining rhetoric, but it also requires the researcher to attend to the cultural mediations of "mothering." For example, does the continual use of the term impose a moral order on faculty members that would not apply if they were simply defined as instructors and not also kin, or even "children"? Do the culturally associated sentiments of the term serve to articulate interpersonal obligations and call out feelings relating, say, to infractions, that go way beyond those that might ensue from simple intellectual disagreements. For instance, a faculty member may disagree with the Department chair on what constitutes a passable examination and, to that extent, produce the sense that there is a difference in perspective. But to disagree with a chair who also "mothers" her faculty also risks feelings of filial betrayal. In other words, the cultural configurations, associated sentimental expectations, and interactive burdens of an interpretive vocabulary condition the construction and applications of the familial as a term of reference.

This is precisely what Harvey Sacks (1992) had in mind when he lectured about *membership categorization devices*. Sacks pointed out that, in practice, terms of reference are not applied willy nilly in everyday life, nor do they arbitrarily relate to what we do and feel in response to them. Rather, terms are membership categorization devices in that they work to inform us of recognizable connections and courses of action, and even how we should feel in response to their application. Now, of course, we may choose to act differently and to feel otherwise, but as cultural configurations–with their shared cognitive and affective linkages–they categorize what we do and who we are as members of a communicative body and, in that sense, organize our relationships. As Sacks might put it, for example, the term "mother" *works* to organize our relationships and their associated actions and sentiments. The constructionist's sensitivity to the cultural conditioning of language use reins in the sense that "anything goes," focusing the researcher's attention on the social organization and accountability of usage.

There are, of course, many conditions that mediate interpretive practice, that circumscribe the application of familial terminology, not the least of which are the local institutional discourses we discussed earlier. Taken together, these cultural and institutional sources provide an important set of ordering contexts that shape the construction process. The methodological imperative, then, is for constructionist researchers to seek out and document artful family-constructing practices, but also to be attentive to the circumstances that condition interpretation.

Substantive Concerns

The constructionist approach to family has also led some to ask if there can be any *concrete* sense of family from this perspective. Is the substance of family displaced by its vocabulary and associated rhetorics? Does the constructionist approach do away with any semblance of the family as a real object of social life? Is it possible for the constructionist researcher to document *how* family and associated realities are constructed while still respecting the sense in which they are "real" working entities of everyday life?

One way of addressing these substantive questions is to engage in the procedural operation called "analytic bracketing" (Gubrium & Holstein, 1997). In order to make visible the constitutive process by which social forms are given a semblance of reality, one must temporarily set aside belief in their substantive existence. Phenomenologists, ethnomethodologists, and other constructionists typically suspend belief in the reality of things in order to render their production visible. Put simply, the *whats* of social life are temporarily put on hold as a way of getting a clearer picture of *how* things (meanings) are accomplished.

This does not mean that the meaningfully real does not exist for constructionists; it is only temporarily suspended as an operating assumption for analytic purposes. Actually, constructionists are more, not less, concerned with the substantive reality of the familial than are other theorists of family life. Indeed, the very substance of the familial is constructionists' empirical stock in trade. Constructionists do not take the reality of family for granted. They don't simply assume that there is "a" traditional family form, for example, but look to see how *the* family is discursively or ideologically asserted (Bernardes, 1985, 1993, 1997; Cheal, 1991; Smith, 1993). They refuse to believe that family demographics straightforwardly represent "family" composition and organization (Cicourel, 1974). They do not ignore the varied and sundry applications of the term, which can extend to remote and obscure nooks and crannies of daily life, far removed from conventional domains of domesticity (Gubrium & Holstein, 1990). They search for *the* family–as a matter of everyday usage–in courtrooms, counseling centers, support groups, nursing homes, schools, on television talk shows, indeed anywhere that family is made topical as a going concern (Gubrium & Holstein, 1987).

The use of bracketing presents the family and other social forms as remarkable realities, things quite worthy of notice. What are otherwise routine social objects may be transformed into objects of inquiry, leading researchers to ask how, and from what, they attain their substantiality? For example, how is it that a legal entity called a family is experienced by members as "no family at all" (Gubrium & Holstein, 1990), while a circle of friends can be "tight as sisters" (Stack, 1974)? How is it that family in one setting is actually detected in the way family members arrange themselves while seated in a counselor's waiting room, while in another setting family is more directly perceived in how members communicate with one another (Gubrium,

1992)? Such questions suggest a radically empirical concern with the substance of the familial and how it is talked into being. The aim of constructionist family studies is to describe that substance of family life and document how it achieves its sense of substantiality.

If the substantive reality of the familial is revealed through the study of related talk and interaction, we might also ask what is the social distribution of family discourse and other related talk in contemporary life? Is it limited to households, to the so-called private sphere? Where and when does family terminology–with its related social forms such as mother, father, child, and grandparent–and its classically connected sentiments–filial responsibility, parental respect, or family loyalty, for example–get talked about? In his book *The History of Sexuality, Volume 1*–which is as much about intimate relations in general as it is about sexual life–Foucault (1980) argues that the private sphere began to take on its varied substances and forms as these matters became topics of public discourse in the 18th and 19th centuries. More recently, Anthony Giddens (1992) argues that what he calls "plastic sexuality" is the product of what has become an intimacy industry, in which the substance of sexuality, love, and the erotic are not only up for open viewing in the media, but bought or otherwise paid for in myriad clinics and therapeutic agencies.

The upshot of this deprivatization of the familial is a virtual explosion, not a diminution, of family (Gubrium & Holstein, 1990; Holstein & Gubrium, 1995). Family and its related social forms are everywhere in contemporary life and its current discourses, informing our politics, our senses of domesticity, the ways we experience relationships, our orientations to interpersonal responsibility, even the rhetoric and accounts we use to make claims about ourselves. Linked in this way with a concern for the discourses of experience, constructionists do not abandon family as an object of social life. Instead, they help us to see just how much the private, family sphere occupies our attention in contemporary times. From the constructionist point of view, family is more central, more important than ever.

Theoretical Concerns

A third set of concerns regarding the constructionist approach is theoretical. Put simply, some have asked, "Just what kind of theory is this?" Analyzing domestic life and related social forms in terms of interpretive practice calls for a minimalist approach to theorizing. The objective is not to take the familial and/or its varied social forms as independent or dependent variables and formulate models of how these variables relate to one another. Nor is the aim to trace family's institutional, historical, or cultural contours, representing it as a product of particular times or ways of life. These goals, in turn, are certainly not ruled out by and indeed may be combined with a constructionist approach. The foremost concern, however, is to consider how family comes into being originally in an indigenously meaningful sense, even while this is ineluctably tied to institutional, historical, and cultural questions. What is theoretically minimalist about this is the refusal to theorize in relation to "broader" matters that are not well understood or appreciated locally and, as a result, are often taken for granted as realities.

A theoretically minimalist approach orients initially to the phenomenon as a mundane reality (Pollner, 1987), with the focus being on how people "theorize" the familial in everyday life. It doesn't jump into theory on its own, as it were, but provides a space for considering how people–everyday actors–think about, define, categorize, catalog, and assign meaning to their relationships in familial terms. The orientation is concerned with how people *use* theory to make meaning in the ordinary "heres" and "theres" of daily living. The approach minimizes its own theorizing in order to attend to everyday persons' "theory work."

The constructionist approach thus provides a way of theorizing about ordinary theory, about what Melvin Pollner (1987) calls "mundane reason." It is concerned with how members of situations and circumstances apply what they know in order to account for what they do. It examines how persons explain what has happened and is happening to them, and what they expect to come about in the future. Where the social sciences tend to denigrate "commonsense" and to take delight in debunking "what everybody knows," constructionism refuses to dismiss the mundane as so much uninformed or illogical "claptrap." It does not engage in invidious comparisons between what people know, think, or believe, on the one hand, and what is scientifically known, on the other. Rather, the constructionist project is precisely to document ordinary knowledge and explanation in order to gain a sense for, among other things, how the familial is understood by those concerned, how it is seen as entering their lives, and how it is constructed by way of commonsense notions of the domestic.

There is a profound analytic neutrality associated with theoretical minimalism–something akin to what Garfinkel and Sacks (1970) called ethnomethodological indifference. No one is taken to be either right or wrong about what they think family is. No one's explanations of family matters are judged correct or incorrect. Rather, each and every one is viewed as being in command of a set of practical understandings that they use, for better or worse, to assign meaning to their relationships. "Better" or "worse" is determined by them, not us (the analysts/researchers). Evaluation is a feature of indigenous interpretive practice, not an analytic objective. For example, analytically, there are no dysfunctional families, only families that have attained that status because an interested party, or agency, or family members themselves, categorize the family as dysfunctional. Analytically, there are no functional families either; there are only families that have had the status socially conferred upon them, or for whom the status is taken for granted. Only a profound analytic neutrality can reveal indigenous sources of meaning and social order.

The space created by theoretical minimalism and analytic neutrality raises many questions. What are the sources of the familial definitions and categories that people apply to their lives? What areas of experience, if any, are devoid of such application? What local conditions shape the ways familiar definitions and categories are articulated with experience? How do these situations differ? What is the interactional machinery of the familial? How do talk and interaction realize the concrete substance of intimate relations? How and where is application contested? What is the social organization and distribution of family rhetoric? How are rhetoric and reality related to each other in interpretive practice? These are only a few of the questions that might be further developed and extended to broader institutional, historical, and cultural concerns.

Practical Concerns

A fourth and final concern relates to the practical implications of the constructionist approach. What benefit is there in approaching family as a social construction? How does this help (or hinder) our domestic affairs or related social policy?

In general, the approach loosens the conceptual ties between how we talk and think about family life–family's representational forms–and what is taken to be the "reality" of the family. At present, with all the public debate about the sanctity of domestic life, the salience of the "traditional" family, and the importance of preserving family values, the underlying issue seems to be whether "the" family, as a social reality, should be represented by a particular social form or should be assigned meaning in terms of diverse social relationships (including, but not restricted to, so-called traditional arrangements).

The conservatives are on one side, arguing that the connection between reality and representation is not arbitrary, but ought to center on "the" true reality of family life. What that reality is, specifically, depends on one's particular sentiments. For some, this refers to the nuclear family, composed of mother, father, and children. For others, it extends to intergenerational linkages. Typically, "the" reality does not include the growing variety of contemporary alternative life styles.

Liberals are on the other side of the issue. Liberal opinion also centers on "the" reality of family, but differs from conservative views in that it is more willing to embrace a wide variety of living arrangements as properly familial. Thus, family life and family values are seen as expressed in one-parent families, commuter marriages, common law marriages, arrangements of convenience, gay marriages, and so on. The idea here is that familial sentiments and their associated rights and responsibilities define the family, not particular legal or biological ties. For example, liberals might argue that a lesbian marriage that is loving, trusting, and supportive is more of a marriage than a conventional, legal, heterosexual marriage ridden with animosity and interpersonal violence.

Whether conservative or liberal, however, the view is that a domestic or marital reality of some kind anchors what it means to "be family." The constructionist approach does not sit squarely in either camp, but, in its fashion, moves beyond both. Focused as the constructionist approach is on the interpretive practices of family life, the reality of family itself is always problematic. The resulting research questions inquire into diverse positions, both conservative and liberal. Exploring the conservative side, questions arise concerning how "the" reality of the traditional family is assigned its substance and what rhetorical devices are applied to represent "the" family as foundational, even sacred? Peering behind liberal views, one might ask how a common reality–family–is represented in manifold interpersonal relationships and what rhetorical means are used to convince us that there is unity in diversity? In a sense, these are identical questions. Except for their application to opposite ends of the political spectrum, the questions are about the representational status of family rhetoric and, in turn, the substantive embodiment of that which is being represented.

In this regard, the constructionist approach traces family's interpretive practices across political views, searching for and aiming to document how it is that family is assigned meaning and experienced as a social form. Some claim that, in this respect, the approach is apolitical and, therefore, cannot claim to have practical utility or policy applications. We see this differently. Our view, as far as family is concerned, is that there is no "given" relationship between reality and representation. Rather, the relationship is eminently social and contingent, one of our own making. We construct the reality of the familial, whether it be "the" traditional family or an alternative arrangement. We assign meaning to our relationships using culturally recognizable family understandings as resources, but an unmediated reality is not among these. The constructionist view, in effect, levels the playing field, but without necessarily taking sides.

From this, we derive the general benefits of understanding and insight. As a practical matter, we have a basis for understanding how it is that conservatives can warrant universalistic claims to acceptable familial forms. We gain insight into the representational and rhetorical strategies of universalism, their conceptual methodologies and empirical tactics. Similarly, we have grounds for understanding the persuasiveness of liberal representations and can reap the insights of examining parallel liberal representational rhetorical and empirical strategies.

General as this is, it provides footing for assessing the accounts offered for both the traditional and its alternatives. Perhaps more importantly, it offers a vantage point for evaluating social policy options by opening the political debate itself to analysis. Rather than accepting the parameters of debate, it deconstructs them, making transparent the objects of discussion and the rhetorics of their construction, showing how our everyday truths are interpretively secured by our own assumptions, means of communication, and "common" sense of the real. This does not cast doubt on reality, but it does provide a political context for considering its possibilities. In the end, it allows us to make personal, moral choices and decisions without the tyranny of essentialist claims-making.

REFERENCES

Ahrne, G. (1990). *Agency and organization*. London: Sage.

Allen, K. R., & Demo, D. H. (1995). The families of lesbians and gay men: A new frontier in family research. *Journal of Marriage and the Family, 57*, 111-127.

Anderson, E. (1981). *A place on the corner*. Chicago: University of Chicago Press.

Baber, K. M., & Allen, K. R. (1992). *Women and families: Feminist reconstructions*. New York: Guilford.

Baca Zinn, M. (1992). Reframing the revisions: Inclusive thinking for family sociology. In C. Kramarae & D. Spender (Eds.), *The knowledge explosion* (pp. 473-479). New York: Teachers College Press.

Berger, P. L., & Luckmann, T. (1966). *The social construction of reality*. Garden City, New York: Anchor.

Bernardes, J. (1985). "Family ideology": Identification and exploration. *Sociological Review, 33*, 275-297.

Bernardes, J. (1993). Responsibilities in studying postmodern families. *Journal of Family Issues, 14*, 35-49.

Bernardes, J. (1999). We must not define "the family"! *Marriage and Family Review* (this volume).

Boss, P., Doherty, W. G., LaRossa, R., Schumm, W. R. & Steinmetz, S. K. (Eds.). (1993). *Sourcebook of family theories and methods*. New York: Plenum.

Cheal, D. (1991). *Family and the state of theory*. Toronto: University of Toronto Press.

Cheal, D. (1993). Unity and difference in postmodern families. *Journal of Family Issues, 14*, 5-19.

Cicourel, A. V. (1974). *Theory and method in a study of Argentine fertility*. New York: Wiley.

Douglas, M. (1986). *How institutions think*. Syracuse, New York: Syracuse University Press.

Drucker, P. (1993). *Post-capitalist society*. New York: Harper.

Durkheim, E. (1961). *The elementary forms of the religious life*. New York: Free Press.

Foucault, M. (1973). *The birth of the clinic*. New York: Vintage.

Foucault, M. (1979). *Discipline and punish*. New York: Vintage.

Foucault, M. (1980). *The history of sexuality*, (Vol. 1). New York: Vintage.

Garfinkel, H. (1967). *Studies in ethnomethodology*. Englewood Cliffs, NJ: Prentice-Hall.

Garfinkel, H., & Sacks, H. (1970). On formal structures of practical actions. In J. C. McKinney & E. A. Tiryakian (Eds.), *Theoretical sociology* (pp. 338-366). New York: Appleton Century Crofts.

Giddens, A. (1992). *The transformation of intimacy*. Stanford, CA: Stanford University Press.

Gubrium, J. F. (1987). Organizational embeddedness and family life. In T. Brubaker (Ed.) *Aging, health and family* (pp. 23-41). Newbury Park, CA: Sage.

Gubrium, J. F. (1989). Local cultures and service policy. In J. F. Gubrium & D. Silverman (Eds.), *The politics of field research* (pp. 94-112). London: Sage.

Gubrium, J. F. (1992). *Out of control: Family therapy and domestic disorder*. Newbury Park, CA: Sage.

Gubrium, J. F., & Holstein, J. A. (1987). The private image: Experiential location and method in family studies. *Journal of Marriage and the Family, 49,* 773-786.

Gubrium, J. F., & Holstein, J. A. (1990). *What is family?* Mountain View, CA: Mayfield.

Gubrium, J. F., & Holstein, J. A. (1993a). Family discourse, organizational embeddedness, and local enactment. *Journal of Family Issues, 14,* 66-81.

Gubrium, J. F., & Holstein, J. A. (1993b). Phenomenology, ethnomethodology, and family discourse. In P. Boss, W. Doherty, R. LaRossa, W. Schumm, & S. Steinmetz (Eds.), *Sourcebook of Family Theory and Methods* (pp. 651-672). New York: Plenum.

Gubrium, J. F., & Holstein, J. A. (1994). Grounding the postmodern self. *The Sociological Quarterly, 35,* 685-708.

Gubrium, J. F., & Holstein, J. A. (1995a). Individual agency, the ordinary and postmodern life. *The Sociological Quarterly, 36,* 701-716.

Gubrium, J. F., & Holstein, J. A. (1995b). Qualitative inquiry and the deprivatization of experience. *Qualitative Inquiry, 1,* 204-222.

Gubrium, J. F., & Holstein, J. A. (1997). *The new language of qualitative method*. New York: Oxford University Press.

Heritage, J. (1984). *Garfinkel and ethnomethodology*. Cambridge, UK: Polity Press.

Holstein, J. A. (1988). Studying "family usage": Family image and discourse in mental hospitalization decisions. *Journal of Contemporary Ethnography, 17,* 261-284.

Holstein, J. A. (1993). *Court-ordered insanity: Interpretive practice and involuntary commitment*. Hawthorne, New York: Aldine de Gruyter.

Holstein, J. A., & Gubrium, J. F. (1994a). Constructing family: Descriptive practice and domestic order. In T. Sarbin & J. Kitsuse (Eds.) *Constructing the social* (pp. 232-250). London: Sage.

Holstein, J. A., & Gubrium, J. F. (1994b). Phenomenology, ethnomethodology, and interpretive practice. In N. Denzin & Y. Lincoln (Eds.) *Handbook of Qualitative Research* (pp. 262-272). Newbury Park, CA: Sage.

Holstein, J. A., & Gubrium, J. F. (1995). Deprivatization and the construction of domestic life. *Journal of Marriage and the Family, 57,* 894-908.

Hopper, J. (1993). The rhetoric of motives in divorce. *Journal of Marriage and the Family, 55,* 801-813.

Lasch, C. (1977). *Haven in a heartless world.* New York: Basic Books.

Levin, I. (1993). Family as mapped realities. *Journal of Family Issues, 14,* 82-91.

Marx, K. (1964). *Selected works in sociology and social philosophy.* New York: Macmillan.

McLain, R., & Weigert, A. (1979). Toward a phenomenological sociology of the family: A programmatic essay. In W. Burr, R. Hill, F. I. Nye, & I. Reiss (Eds.), *Contemporary theories about the family* (Vol. 2, pp. 160-205). New York: Free Press.

Miller, G. (1991). Family as excuse and extenuating circumstance: Social organization and use of family rhetoric in a work incentive program. *Journal of Marriage and the Family, 53,* 609-21.

Miller, L. J. (1990a). Safe home, dangerous street: Remapping social reality in the early modern era. In G. Miller & J. Holstein (Eds.), *Perspectives on social problems,* (Vol. 2, pp. 45-66). Greenwich, CT: JAI Press.

Miller, L. J. (1990b). Violent families and the rhetoric of harmony. *British Journal of Sociology, 41,* 263-88.

Pollner, M. (1987). *Mundane reason.* New York: Cambridge University Press.

Presthus, R. L. (1978). *The organizational society.* New York: St. Martin's.

Rosenblatt, P. C. (1994). *Metaphors for the family.* New York: Guilford.

Rosenblatt, P. C., & Fischer, L. R. (1993). Qualitative family research. In P. Boss, W. Doherty, R. LaRossa, W. Schumm, & S. Steinmetz (Eds.), *Sourcebook of Family Theories and Methods* (pp. 167-177). New York: Plenum.

Sacks, Harvey. (1992). *Lectures on conversation* (Vol. 1 & 2). Cambridge, MA: Blackwell.

Schutz, A. (1970). *On phenomenology and social relations.* Chicago: University of Chicago Press.

Smith, D. E. (1993). The Standard North American Family: SNAF as an ideological code. *Journal of Family Issues, 14,* 50-65.

Stacey, J. (1990). *Brave new families.* New York: Basic Books.

Stack, C. (1974). *All our kin.* New York: Harper & Row.

Thompson, L. (1992). Feminist methodology for family studies. *Journal of Marriage and the Family, 54,* 3-18.

Walker, A. J. (1993). Teaching about race, gender, and class diversity in United States families. *Family Relations, 42,* 342-350.

We Must Not Define "The Family"!

Jon Bernardes

INTRODUCTION

In addressing the question of "What is Family?" it is important to note that most sociologists take the response to such a question as being quite straightforward. Most sociologists would miss the subtlety of the question "What is Family?" and proceed to take the existence of "The Family" as an absolute taken-for-granted idea; much grand theorizing actually depends upon the presumed existence and character of "The Family" (Bernardes, 1985a). Less related to grand theory and more to contemporary right-wing political positions, there are those in the United Kingdom who argue very fiercely that "The Family" does exist (Anderson & Dawson, 1986; Durham, 1985; Fitzgerald, 1983). These interests even appear to suggest that "it" is in some kind of crisis and should be supported at all costs. Such authors tend to argue against variation and diversity in family life as being "deviant" or "pathological."

Cheal (1991) examines four strategies used to handle family changes. Under *Concept Specification*, he discusses approaches such as that of Nave-Herz who accepts that there may be significant contemporary changes in family forms. He continues to assert, however, that "The Family" is culturally universal and thus a focus of theorizing and investigation. Under *Concept Abandonment*, he explores Scanzoni's attempt to escape from the limitations of "The Family" by focusing on close relationships and primary relationships. In *Concept Displacement*, Cheal explores those he labels as Post-positivist theorists such as myself and Gubrium and Holstein; who "do not try to escape from lay concepts of reality, but rather attempt to confront them

Jon Bernardes is affiliated with the University of Wolverhampton, Castle View, Dudley, West Midlands, DY1 3HR, UK.

[Haworth co-indexing entry note]: "We Must Not Define 'The Family'!" Bernardes, Jon. Co-published simultaneously in *Marriage & Family Review* (The Haworth Press, Inc.) Vol. 28, No. 3/4, 1999, pp. 21-41; and: *Concepts and Definitions of Family for the 21st Century* (ed: Barbara H. Settles et al.) The Haworth Press, Inc., 1999, pp. 21-41. Single or multiple copies of this article are available for a fee from The Haworth Document Delivery Service [1-800-342-9678, 9:00 a.m. - 5:00 p.m. (EST). E-mail address: getinfo@ haworthpressinc.com].

directly, within social theory" (Cheal, 1991, p. 130). In simpler terms, Post-positivists reject the existence of "The Family" in concrete reality and focus instead upon the construction, use, location and power of the term in every-day language or contemporary discourse. In *Concept Expansion*, he locates the work of Trost and the Rapoports. The Rapoports accept the widespread diversity of family life but focus instead upon a generalized model of diversi-ty within an understanding of "The Family" (Rapoport, & Rapoport, 1977, 1982). Trost (1988) has clearly argued that "there is no possibility of defining the family" (p. 301), but develops a model of "family" in terms of parent-child and spousal units. Trost (1990) notes: "Evidently no-one 'knows' what a family is: our perspectives vary to such a degree that to claim to know what a family is shows a lack of knowledge" (p. 442). Everyday actors do have meanings for the term "The Family"; our job is not to abstract and crystallise these–such an approach is bound to lead to reification. Rather our job, as Gubrium and Holstein (1990) say so often, is to study how actors generate and sustain such meanings.

An increasing number of researchers are using terms such as "family," "family life," "families" instead of "The Family" (Doherty & Campbell, 1988; Gubrium & Holstein, 1990; Zinn & Eitzen, 1990). The issue of defin-ing "The Family" could be relegated to a student exercise if it were not for our general pre-occupation with the problems of family life such as divorce, child rearing, or child sexual abuse (Feminist Review, 1988). A great deal of the analysis of such family problems is couched in terms of the "decline" or "collapse" of "The Family." It is only by grasping that "The Family" does not exist, that the ideological nature of such analyses can be recognized.

This issue is important to sociology because each and every time a sociol-ogist (or anyone else) utters the term "The Family" they act upon society (Bernardes, 1987). Their words have not only meaning but substance in that they are literally "Doing Things with Words" (Gubrium & Lynott, 1985). Such words can and do change people's lives or reinforce certain patterns of behavior. In some cases, the users of such terms would approve of the results of their words; approve of consigning women to mothering roles; approve of freeing men from domestic tasks even when they are in the home; approve of condemning to silence the vast majority of parents and spouses who, from time to time, find themselves fighting a losing battle to maintain the appear-ance of normality in sexuality, parenting, marriage, etc. (Durham, 1985; Fitzgerald, 1983; Anderson & Dawson, 1986).

The idea of "The Family" or "The Nuclear Family" is an idea with remark-able strength and power. It is something which just about any member of society can offer a definition of and which many powerful lobbies (politics, morality, religion) claim to support and revere. The image of "The Family" is quite clear, as Segal (1983:13) suggests:

Our traditional family model of the married heterosexual couple with children–based on a sexual division of labour where the husband as breadwinner provides economic support for his dependent wife and children, while the wife cares for both husband and children–remains central to all family ideology.

Ordinary people generally miss the difference between "family" and "The Family" and revert all too readily to the image of "The Nuclear Family" that features so large in many European societies. The simplest but also most serious problem that researchers in this area have to contend with is that of communicating with colleagues and lay persons.

VARIATION AND DIVERSITY IN FAMILIES

We need to ask whether the extent of variation and diversity is important enough to invalidate the idea of "The Nuclear Family." The many and varied features that make families in any way "different" from the ideal model all count as variation, and in that consideration "The Nuclear Family" does not exist except as a powerful image in the minds of most people.

In exploring a "Framework for Family Studies," Weeks (1986) summarizes the efforts of Rapoport and Rapoport (1977; 1982) to identify five types of diversity.

1. *Organizational Diversity in Families.* Primarily a result of diverse patterns of internal domestic labour or patterns of working outside the family home. This form of diversity will be influenced by the extent and nature of unpaid work within a family.

2. *Cultural Diversity in Families.* There are very clear, but often completely neglected, variations in behaviors, beliefs and practices as a result of culture, ethnicity, political and religious affiliations. It is important to realize that there may be very wide variations within white groups just as there are wide variations within and between a wide range of "non-white" groups.

3. *Social Class Diversity in Families.* There are obvious variations resulting from marked differences in the availability of material and social resources. These will range from simply having enough food, to attitudes towards whether infants should be reared by their mothers or paid "Nannies," or whether or not children should be sent away to boarding schools.

4. *Cohort Diversity in Families.* It is clear that particular historical periods mean that people born within that period will have quite different experiences from those born in different periods. The obvious cases are

periods of war and civil disruption, such as the "Troubles" in Northern Ireland, and less clear historically located events across Europe, such as increases in divorce, single parenthood and cohabitation.

5. *Family Life Course Diversity.* This form recognizes how life changes dramatically with events in the course of life, for example, having children, whether a child is a baby or teenager. Having said this, it is vital to recognize that the other four forms of diversity mean that it is extremely unlikely that all families will pass through "essentially similar" phases. It is not likely, for example, that a poor African Caribbean couple having their first child will have the same experiences as a wealthy public-school educated couple. Similarly, within similar levels of wealth and resources, it is unlikely that a dual working nominally Christian couple will have the same experiences as a male-breadwinner, orthodox Jewish couple.

At a more detailed level there are many things that make families special: wealth, housing, transportation, poverty, age, death, disability, unemployment, ethnicity, education, paid work, whether both parents work, number of children, twins or multiple births. Are babies different from toddlers or teenagers? Are all couples much the same or do they merely appear much the same until they split up? Are all husbands breadwinners? Are all wives homemakers? Are we all always fit and healthy? Does sickness or disability make a difference? Do parents always love each other and their children? Do children always get along with their parents or other children in their family? Do we all have similar hopes, ideals, and interests? Are we all decently non-violent? What about domestic murder, child abuse and child sexual abuse? What about the shared private worlds of sexual behavior or the even more private individual worlds of innermost thoughts, beliefs and secrets?

In 1967, Mayer (1967a) argued that we are likely to know surprisingly little about the married lives of other people because the greater part of marriage is unseen or invisible. Mayer later suggested that the invisibility of marriage and family life results from the "assumptive world" within which we operate (1967b). We do not need to see the marriages of other people because we make assumptions about what goes on within marriage or "family."

Marriage and family life are intensely private affairs in contemporary societies. Ball (1975) related deviance to the degree of privacy, noting that the more private an area of behavior is, the more likely there are to be clear public social norms and extensive private deviance. All such family problems are seen as outside the model of "The Family" and therefore as deviant or abnormal.

Evidence that "The Family" model may not match the reality of "family life" generates calls to uphold that very model of "The Family." Sociology has lent credibility to the idea of "The Family" and has, as so many feminists have observed (Oakley, 1974, 1981, 1982a, 1982b; Beechey, 1985; Barrett, 1980), tended to support conservative, right-wing ideas. To continue this pattern of defining "family" will perpetuate the wholesale oppression of men, women and children–in short, the whole of society.

Sociology and psychology have testified to the universality and naturalness of "The Family" (Collier, 1982), the biological imperative of the division of the sexes (Wilson, 1975; Rossi, 1977), and the rejection as "unnatural" of all variant family forms (Sussman, 1973, 1975; Anderson & Dawson, 1986; Whitfield, 1987). If "The Family" is natural and universal, then people who fail to convince themselves that their own situation is a case of "The Family," are likely to label themselves as unnatural. Moreover, the image of universality encourages many people to try to make their own family life like the image of "The Family" and imitate what may be uncomfortable and unworkable images of personal behavior and gender. It is astonishing the impact sociology has had on society in glorifying and continually extolling "The Family," in the oppression of huge numbers of individuals and the creation of suffering and misery on a truly grand scale (Bernardes, 1985b, 1986a, 1986b, 1987, 1988).

To confront such oppression, I have engaged in a series of explorations of theoretical issues surrounding family life. There are major problems. First, most people will not accept that "The Family" does not exist; even those who accept variation and diversity still want to use the ideal-type model as some kind of standard or measure. Second, most people simply refuse to consider the central ideological location of the image of "The Family" and the practice of "family life." Third, until a range of recent methodological developments, there has been no other way of looking at family life except through the framework of an ideal-type. Fourth, this refusal to acknowledge variation and diversity has generated a family policy that may be seriously damaging to many citizens.

Counting "The Family"

Very few scholars have ever bothered to ask if "The Family" exists or ever has existed. In 1925, Bowley and Hogg found that the conventional family (of a wage-earning man, his wife and three dependent children) accounted for only 5% of all families in the Northern counties of the United Kingdom. Using 1978 Government statistics, Rapoport and Rapoport (1982) found that only 20% of UK households contained single-breadwinner families. Rimmer and Wicks (1981) argued that such a family type only accounted for 15% of households. Westwood (1984) noted that such a model represented only 5% of UK households. In the United States, Ramey (1978) found that only 13% of families corresponded to the nuclear family model of father as sole breadwinner with mother at home rearing the children. There have been few estimates since, but in 1989, Ricketts and Achtenberg (1989) claimed that only 7% of the US population lived in such a situation.

Analysis based on the 1981 UK Census suggested that less than 2% of families corresponded to the nuclear family model. This takes no account of chronic illness, stage of child rearing, behavioral problems and variations (Bernardes, 1986b; Murphy, 1983). Based on the 1991 Census in the UK, there were 21,897,322 households; some 1,503,888 of these households contained one adult male and one adult female with between one and three dependent children where only one of the adults was in employment. This suggests that only 14.6% of households contained this particular household form. This proportion will include, however, unmarried adults, unrelated adults and children, chronically sick persons (some 8% of all age groups), and all the other variations that can be thought of. It seems very likely indeed that the proportion of households matching a stricter definition of "The Nuclear Family" will be a small fraction of one percent (Office of Population Censuses and Surveys, 1992a, 1992b). One common response is to argue that while "The Nuclear Family" may not be in the majority at a particular moment in time, it is nonetheless a "stage" through which all families must pass. While many do pass through a stage in which there are two adults and one or two children, this does not represent a common experience. The outcomes of that particular stage are extremely varied, ranging from abuse and divorce to different types of marriage. The superficial appearance of there being two adults and two children tells us nothing at all about what actually goes on in that stage.

A more basic conceptual flaw reflects a misunderstanding in sociology, that people share common experiences of a given situation, such as women in childbirth or motherhood. Similar, perhaps common, circumstances may exist, but their experiences are varied and diverse. Some will be rich, some poor, some experience postnatal depression, others may be almost euphoric. The first step is to reject the idea of "The Family" by demonstrating that the way people actually live their family lives turns out to be far more complex, varied and diverse than popular stereotypes allow.

The Role of Family Ideology

Many sociologists have failed to recognize the depth and power of family ideology. Notions of "The Family" are embedded in accounts of the biological bases of sexual inequality, explanations of the process of industrial change and a shift from extended to nuclear family types. Given this centrality, it is possible that critical re-evaluations of "The Family" have been largely unthinkable on the part of those whose careers are based in the validity of such theorizing.

Mannheim (1972) distinguished two levels of ideology, the particular and the total. In the particular he identified the kinds of views that might be held by an opponent, where it is possible to express skepticism. In contrast, total ideology meant the ideas of an era or socio-historical group (Mannheim, 1972). In referring to this aspect of family ideology, Morgan (1985) argues that:

> What ideology does, in effect, is to select from the range of possible ways in which a society might handle the relationships between the biological and the cultural, particularly in the sphere of childbirth and parenthood, and to proclaim the method so selected as the method, as natural and inevitable. (p. 295)

Barrett (1980) suggests that ideology is not just a set of abstract ideas but is expressed in everyday actions. This is important as the means by which ideology is reproduced or passed from one person to another and continually reinforced. It is not just that many people think of women as the most appropriate caregivers for children but rather that we all act on this belief in our daily lives. Men may hesitate or not know how to engage in certain tasks or, in public, men may be discouraged from comforting a lost child, while a woman may naturally take up this role. Levin (1990) noted that, "If one has a closed and non-problematicized concept of family, certain types of inter-pretations of social reality are made. . . . The concepts we use decide what we see" (p. 18). Family ideology as supported by family sociology, has ensured that we have paid attention to white, middle-class, two-parent families. Also, some aspects of social existence are simply not seen. For example, modernist family theorizing denied the possibility of widespread abuse or unhappiness in "The Family."

Family ideology plays a vital role in sustaining an individualistic mode of thought. Ribbens (1994) notes how the "core notions of 'the Individual' and 'The Family' can be seen as both polarized and intertwined" (p. 46). Family ideology involves the development of extreme individualism. Being a father is distinct from being a mother; the roles of son or daughter depend upon the age, sex and blood relationships. "The Family" is seen to contain unique positions occupied by individuals. Try and think of a way in which to rear children so that they do not become so extremely individualistic (Ribbens, 1994).

Family ideology supports the way in which we all see ourselves as unique and different. The creation of difference, and inequality, rests upon distin-guishing individuals by the apparently objective facts of age, gender, biologi-cal relationships. It is hardly surprising that many feminists have shown a deep hostility towards "The Family" in that it is an idea that underpins the creation of gender difference and inequality (Barrett & McIntosh, 1991). Family ideology allows us all to deceive ourselves into believing in our own normality by creating and sustaining an image of "The Family." This vagueness means we can each believe that all families are much the same, they are all "normal," and therefore we do not need to explore everyday family living (Bernardes, 1985b).

The Social Construction of Realities

Social construction of realities within family life according to Berger and Kellner's (1971) work suggests that marriage contributes to our sense of certainty and identity. They focus upon language as the medium by which "the social" is constructed, especially in generating a shared sense of reality. Among the conversations available to individuals, marriage occupies a "privileged status among the significant validating relationships for adults in our society" (Berger & Keller, 1971, p. 24). Summarizing this process, Berger and Kellner (1971:28) argue that

> the process is . . . one in which reality is crystallized, narrowed and stabilized. Ambivalences are converted into certainties. Typifications of self and others become settled. Most generally possibilities become facticities. What is more, the process of transformation remains, most of the time, unapprehended by those who are both its authors and its objects.

Backett (1982) emphasizes human interaction in "family life as a mutually created shared reality" (p. 35), Askham (1984:183) concludes that "marriage is in many ways a compromise between stability-maintaining and identity-upholding behavior, and that on the whole married people perform this balancing act very skillfully." Our first and most important experiences occur within, and are largely determined by, family life.

The way in which realities and ideologies are constructed within family life effectively mystifies our own lives. Not only are certain practices presented as real to us but alternatives are also closed off as unnatural. The process of the social construction of realities and ideologies that I have experienced has structured my relationships with other human beings in ways that I cannot avoid or deny.

Social Structure

The final theoretical aspect of studying family lives concerns the most basic of sociological concerns: social structure. The questions are "how is society possible?" and "what enables us to occupy a place within society?" Is family life the key in constituting social structure and maintaining social order? Within family living the social construction of realities presents to us: people, power, inequality, love and obligations as real. In structuring our most basic relationships with parents, siblings, lovers, children and kin, family living serves to instruct us in the conduct of personal relationships. Family ideology structures human relationships in age and gender and the wider dimensions of power, authority, deference and respect (Bernardes, 1985b). In establishing the pattern of parental authority, "The Family" serves as a basic instruction for many later relationships in education, work, dealings with bureaucracies and citizenship more widely.

Most accounts of social structure emphasize the way actors recognize one another, interact and even co-operate. The hidden structure of fear and intimidation keeps us all in certain locations at certain times or leads us to avoid certain locations at certain times. Family life relates to our own sense of "who we are" and how we "fit into" the lives of others. Critical analysis of family lives inevitably involves examining our beliefs about ourselves (which we usually call reality), our beliefs about others (which we often call ideology), our position in society (location) and the nature of society itself (or social structure).

The concept of "The Family" is rarely regarded as being problematic in itself. Despite the recognition of family diversity, nearly all discussions become a straightforward attack upon, or defense of, "The Family." Gubrium and Holstein (1990:155) argue that their approach "suggests a direction, a new program for "family studies." The key to their approach is the recognition that "the family" is "as much idea as thing" (p. 163). At the pivot of this duality is the simple point that "It is practice that unifies ideas and things" (p. 157).

A preliminary step must be a brief review of the location of family ideology in contemporary society. Most simply stated, the contemporary dominant ideology appears to involve, among others, three specific and mutually reinforcing ideologies: family ideology, gender ideology, and work or wage labor ideology. These three ideologies reflect basic contemporary divisions; the division of the public and the private; the division of the sexes; and, the division of labor.

Perhaps "family ideology" (and NOT "The Family") functions to sustain industrial societies and modes of thought appropriate to industrial societies by means of four key elements. First, family ideology plays a vital role in sustaining an individualistic mode of thought in contemporary societies. Second, family ideology sustains an essentially naturalistic analysis of human behavior. Third, family ideology facilitates and sustains major forms of differentiation in contemporary society. Fourth, and perhaps most contentiously, family ideology constitutes an idolistic mystification of human social life; that is to say that family ideology creates and venerates an idol of "The Family" which mystifies the reality of so-called "family life" (Bernardes, 1985b).

ALTERNATIVE THEORETICAL FRAMEWORKS

The term "post modern family life" was developed by Stacey "to signal the contested, ambivalent, and undecided character of contemporary gender and kinship arrangements" (Stacey, 1990:17). Family Sociology has been deeply positivist in the traditional, natural-science-based approach in the social sciences that assumes the existence of facts, stability and order, and which seeks to be objective and detached. The assumption is that everything is external, "out there." The world is external, objective, factual and requires technical expertise from us to capture, analyze, describe and explain it. Usually, positivism places a heavy emphasis also on rationality and the idea of the purpose or function of behavior and institutions.

Post modernism has developed tools and approaches that seek to understand family lives in new ways, perhaps most easily thought of as looking at family lives "in here" (in our heads). Cheal (1991:5) characterizes post modernism as "an approach that engages in skeptical reflection on the culture of modern society or, in other words, modernity and its dominant world view, namely modernism." In exploring what might be involved in a sociology of the post modern families, Cheal argues that "Post modernist thought in sociology begins from contemporary experiences of pluralism, disorder and fragmentation, which were not predicted by the modern paradigm of universal reason" (p. 9).

A neat example of the insights that can be gained from adopting a post modern perspective comes from a recent study by DeVault (1991) who looks at the role of cooking and meals in the construction of families. Taking a modernist account, the role of the mother in preparing meals is taken for granted and, consequently, very few sociologists have even looked at the topic, though it is a daily experience for the vast majority of families. From a post modernist frame, DeVault is able to demonstrate how the interaction around meals serves to develop and reinforce sex role and age related behaviors between children and parents.

The enormous power of modernist family theorizing can be seen in family discourse. Cheal (1991:20) summarizes this area:

> Social Scientific . . . concepts of "the family," are commonly derived from folk models. . . . When these categories become objects of attention in discussions and debates they acquire common meanings within a shared way of talking, or discourse.

The focus, therefore, is to examine the models people have in their heads and their shared language.

Several scholars have sought to avoid the problem of assuming a model of the typical family by avoiding the idea of "The Family" altogether and using, instead, the concept of household. In pioneering work in 1967, Bender argued that a household may be thought of as a "residence group that carries out domestic functions" while "'a family' should be seen as essentially a kinship group" (p. 493). Ball (1972:302) proposed the adoption of the concept of living together to signal a "cohabiting domestic relationship which is (or has been) sexually consequential." That is, such relationships involve sexual activity and possibly the birth of children, arguing that this approach is "one which says nothing about families *per se* . . . " (p. 302). As a result, this strategy is likely to yield new insights into family living, without imposing sociological definitions about what is or is not "a family" or "The Family."

In the intervening period, the concept of household has come to be adopted by a wide range of researchers to pursue pragmatic research aims. Several feminists have worked on the distribution of resources within households, obtaining important data about gender inequalities in control over resources (Brannen & Wilson, 1987). Most recently, Buck and Scott (1994) have provided the first report of the Research Centre on Micro-Social Change into The British Household Panel Survey. Simply replacing the concept of "family" with that of "household" has not generated new or radical reinterpretations of the nature of family living.

Concepts of household and family are quite distinct in everyday thought and language; the head of household and the head of family may overlap but are different ideas. Gershuny et al. (1994:16) argue that household is an important structure in everyday life but is not the same as "family," noting:

> For most people, at most points in time, there is some small group, which includes one or more other person, which is the principal unit for organization for economic life (in the broadest sense) and the primary channel for emotional expression and biological reproduction. This unit is often the family (i.e., two or more individuals with some current kinship, marital or quasi-marital relation).

In this sense, adopting the term "household" instead of "family" runs all the risks of simply re-importing another popular concept that is not primarily designed for sociological analysis. A great deal of the sentiment and related sense of connection, exchange and obligation goes well beyond the household. Much of the debate about family obligations is about people caring for people in other households (Finch, 1989). The notion of household does not enable analysts to study how people use family language, such as "a good father" or "not really a family." Instead, it is likely that such ordinary everyday language holds the key to understanding how powerful the ideas are that focus on family living.

One important and productive approach has been that of studying the "life courses" of individuals, that is the way our lives develop and change along with personal events such as marriage, the birth of a child or death of a partner. Cohen (1987) speaks of the individual life course as "like a bus journey, with boarding and embarkation points . . . these stages are not fixed" (p. 3). This has, for example, enabled researchers to focus more on dilemmas about returning to paid work at stages in the life course for women or the issue of middle age. In the UK, this approach usually focuses upon individuals, life courses within assumed models of the normal "nuclear family."

In an attempt to facilitate the study of family life, I developed the idea of conceptualizing the coming together of individual life courses upon *Family Pathways* (Bernardes, 1986a). We should think of individual life courses meeting, sometimes being or becoming interdependent, even combining and perhaps later parting. An individual is not merely born nor simply becomes older. An individual occupies and moves through different structures relating to, for example, being a baby, a child, a teenager, a single adult, a spouse, a parent including many important "rites of passage." At all times the individual has to negotiate a pathway through these structures. In exploring mothering, Ribbens (1994:166) argues that

> the everyday experience of bringing up children in family units requires a constant and subtle negotiation to achieve some balance, and the responsibility for this balancing act is largely the mother's, as primary mediator within the family.

Whoever takes the major responsibility, it is clear that all family members are continually negotiating their own pathways.

Another viewpoint is that such life courses and pathways link families to other subsystems of the community. This model allows us to escape from the static picture of "The Family" for a much richer appreciation of variation and diversity. The model of *Family Pathways* is about treating the everyday usage as a proper subject in itself rather than substitute a new sociological concept. With this model, we can look at how people express ideas of family, which may or may not include those outside their households, especially parents and extended kin. It is important to add that an individual's life course is multidimensional and can be sensibly seen in terms of, say, health, education, career, hobbies, sport, etc. Individuals may be party to several pathways with other and perhaps differing sets of individuals. A child may relate to mother, father, or siblings, but may also develop an important shared pathway with a group of teenage contemporaries.

Groups of individuals whose life-courses coincide on the same pathway may refer to themselves as "a family" for some time. Researchers must ask at what point and why people refer to situations as "family." The most obvious situation is where the term "The Family" is used by an individual to refer simultaneously to a small unit (perhaps a one-parent situation) as well as a larger grouping of kin (perhaps including non-biologically related aunts and uncles).

Bearing the model of *Family Pathways* in mind presents families as enormously complex and difficult to study. The portrayal is not of ideal types or typical patterns but a sense of the uniqueness of pathways. Many of us find ourselves facing similar experiences, such as parenthood, but come to these events from very different routes and respond quite differently. Nunally (1988:13) suggests that

> most families encounter external or internal stresses at different points in the life span of each member. These stresses vary from one family to another depending on many factors in the environment and the family.

This begins to hint at the enormous richness of variation and diversity in human family living which is precisely the objective of developing alternative theorizing about family lives.

The lesson to be taken from modernist theorizing is that the cultural, religious, professional and personal values embedded in theorizing have long been implicit and denied. Traditional views of "The Family" have been conservative, racist, classist, and heterosexist. In developing new forms of theorizing and a new post modern sociology of family living, a key strategy is that of exploring a wide range of values.

Understanding our ignorance rests on recognizing the error of believing that you can study family life in isolation and the error of believing that such study will have no practical effect. This has several implications for sociology. First, the way we split up features of social life for study (e.g., class, ethnicity, family, education, crime) and fail to look at the essential unity of people's lives. Second, the way we study surface appearances or even presume features to exist (e.g., "The Family") rather than seek underlying actuality: what is actually going on (Bernardes, 1986a).

Our ignorance is largely a result of the failure of many sociologists to come to terms with the issue of values. Sociologists have often denied their role in generating and upholding particular value positions. In the case of the study of "The Family," the strength and power of values adopted by largely white male sociologists is extremely clear. What was presented as a simple, objective description contained within it wide ranging values relating to the superiority of paid work and the inferiority of women and children. There is no such thing as a value-free sociologist nor can there be a piece of sociological research that is entirely free from human values (Shipman, 1981). There is no such thing as a value-free natural scientist. The search for objectivity and value-freeness is an illusion; merely labeling used by authority to give credibility to some ideas while discrediting other ideas.

Compared to those who design, manufacture and sell intentionally and unintentionally harmful technology, our job in sociology is much more dangerous. People can choose to use science and technology to pollute the world, wage war, oppress or imprison. What we deal in, ideas themselves, are the bases upon which people make choices, including those of polluting the world, waging war, oppressing or imprisoning others. The responsibility is awesome and many might say we are best to deny or avoid this responsibility. We have been doing this for decades, and have wreaked havoc and harm in people's lives.

Sociologists are widely known for being political. Like many sociologists, I detest gross inequality, especially when it is visited upon the weak and innocent (such as the young and the old). At the same time, I recognize that a considerable amount of sociology has failed to recognize that many people support that inequality. In a wider sense, we must recognize that human beings are extremely complex and often contradictory. It is not obvious, for example, that revealing widespread abuse and violence will be well received. Put most simply, if family abuse is widespread then many of our audience will be both abusers and survivors and it will be in their interests to deny or downplay the research. This, of course, is precisely what has happened in the recent decades of exploring forms of family abuse and is the reason abuse is still seen as deviant or abnormal. It is therefore possible that "new understandings" of family life will be significantly liberating. It must be remembered, however, that "changed understandings" risk creating damage and harm.

DEVELOPING A NEW FAMILY STUDIES

As mentioned previously, while *Family Studies* does not exist in the UK, it is a common discipline in the USA, Europe and Australia. Much of what goes under the label of *Family Studies* draws heavily upon the modernist tradition and seeks to find solutions to particular family problems or, indeed, problem families. In recent years, however, a small number of authors, from widely different backgrounds, have made pleas to develop a new form of *Family Studies*.

In 1988, Wesley Burr and his colleagues argued that:

We believe that the family realm has a much greater effect on the human condition than most people realize, and if more of us were to realize that our field is a basic discipline that deals with a profoundly important part of the human condition, it may help us usher in a period of unusual creativity in the next several decades. (p. 205)

Burr et al. (1988) attempted to lay down a definition of the "family realm" to establish "family science." While I do not agree with their particular formulation, I do agree about the centrality of family life.

This article has a clear mission, stating the case for the establishment of a post modern *Family Studies* in the United Kingdom and laying down the essential components of this new discipline in the United Kingdom (Bernardes, 1997). Parties of all kinds have common interests in family life. All agree that people should be given every chance to best prepare themselves for marriage and parenthood. It is in all our interests to support and enhance marriage and parenting. Further generations are vital to us all; the happiness of current generations is also vital to us all. The happiness and well-being of spouses, parents and children must be a prime goal for us all. It is our task to understand how to minimize the pain, suffering and misery of family life and how to maximize the joy, pleasure and love of family life.

Family Citizenship

Because modernist family sociology contributed to a widespread family ideology, it was taking a distinct political stance and contributing to a definition of "The Family" as a political entity. In developing a post modern study of family lives referred to as *Family Studies*, it is important to replace this political entity in an explicit and open fashion. For the present purposes, the notion of *Family Citizenship* will be adopted to replace a central political notion of "The Family" (Bernardes, 1997).

Donati (1991) reviews a set of commonly recognized "family problems" that have arisen in a period of rising affluence and wealth. He suggests that we need to think not of specific problems but rather that families need to be fully recognized as families. In that context, *Family Citizenship* includes the rights and duties held by individuals (only individuals can hold rights and duties) which are only held because of their status in families. The notion of *Family Citizenship* provides an alternative means to categorize or assess family life based on a more realistic and explicit recognition of the importance of families as families. *Family Citizenship* recognizes and enhances individual citizenship, especially of vulnerable groups such as children or the elderly.

Although we live in increasingly material and individualistically orientated societies that emphasize wage earners over the interests of non-earners (children, many women, the aged) or families, the concept of *Family Citizenship* presents a means by which to locate and understand individual rights and obligations in the context of family living rather than in isolation. Recognizing the role of all individuals vis-à-vis families is a significant step towards equality between all individuals. If we are much clearer about rights, duties and obligations of all family members, this may well enhance the position and status of children by recognizing their rights not in abstract isolation (to a decent childhood) but rather in relational location (the need for society to facilitate the provision by parents of a decent childhood).

Much work has been done upon the nature of family obligations that place so many women in a situation of delivering care (Finch, 1989). What is of greatest importance here is to recognize that these distributive patterns are not solely a product of gender but rather conditional upon gender and location in "families." We do not expect just any woman to care for any elderly or disabled person but do expect a wife or daughter to take up the task if she is at all able to do so.

Families are the means whereby material goods (such as food, shelter, transport, money) are distributed to the majority of the population who are not economically active (children and the old, also, women). Much more than this, though, is the distribution of non-material goods centered around the caring relationship–the most obvious cases are in provision of care (often by women) for men, children, the sick and elderly. Segal (1983:9) has typified images of family living as compromises between "love, intimacy, stability, safety, security, privacy . . . (and) . . . fears of abandonment, chaos, failure." It is important to note that while families distribute "goods" such as love, care, nurturance, there has always been significant evidence that they also distribute "bads" such as anger, hate, despair, abuse, or violence. This may go a considerable distance toward clarifying what is sometimes called a "transmission" of behaviors or circumstances such as poverty or abuse. Such social conditions are not genetically inherited but part of the distribution and exchange systems of families.

Many family agendas include a special appeal for the care or nurturance of children. While perfectly reasonable, if taken too far, such an emphasis can generate inequalities between generations where more resources are commanded by the elderly meaning that fewer resources are available for children (Donati, 1991). Already there is a growing concern that the rapidly rising number of elderly people in Europe is diverting scarce resources from caring for our children. Critical work has identified the potential individualism arising out of excessive child-centeredness (Bjornberg, 1992) as well as evidence emerging from China concerning the notion of "child emperors" following the imposition of the "one child" policy. In terms, then, of *Family Citizenship*, families have rights and duties concerning all members with no priorities. If we think in terms of reciprocity and relationships, we should then begin to think about the skills and abilities necessary to engage in relationships. In considering *Family Citizenship*, we should focus upon relationships between all parties rather than insist that one party (say parents) has responsibilities towards others (children).

Family Associations

A final consideration relates to *Family Associations* that Donati described as primary or secondary social networks, with a degree of formal organization, that address the needs of families as families (Bernardes, 1995). They are quite common in other European nations, but distinct from those organizations more familiar in the UK and the USA that tend to focus upon particular aspects of family life such as mothers, children, relationships, or special disability groups. Recent research reveals that there are many small and short-lived voluntary associations that address some part of family living in the UK (Bernardes, 1995). European examples of such associations already possess a wealth of practical experience. The Union of Large and Young Families in the Flemish Community of Belgium boasts several million members out of a population of 7 million; activities include family life education, preparation for childbirth, loans and hire of baby equipment, self-help and mutual support groups for all types of families (single and dual parent), help for the disabled and elderly within families, advice on child rearing and dealing with teenagers. The group promotes solidarity between families, advances the interests of families, and advocates a family and child-orientated society. European family associations may provide valuable models of organization and service delivery.

Some major conferences have debated the nature and shape of social and family policy. In the European Community, this has been part of a move towards a very much more sophisticated policy development process. The European Community has set up what it calls the "European Family Policy Observatory" in which a group of national experts monitor changes in "family life" and make sets of recommendations as to how to develop family policy to meet and accommodate these changes (Bernardes, 1991). Rather than impose family policy on the basis of an abstract model, the trend is to establish what family life is like and attempt to tailor family policy to fit the trends.

In conclusion, three theorems are presented:

1. *Theorem of Sociological Principle.* We must reject entirely the concept of "The Family" as theoretically adequate and, as a consequence, recognize the enormous difficulty, in principle, of studying what actors refer to as "family life." (Bernardes, 1988, p. 72)
2. *Theorem of Sociological Practice.* We must commit ourselves to studying the UNITY of everyday ACTUAL experience and, as a consequence, recognize the enormous difficulty, in practice, of studying what actors refer to as "family life." (Bernardes, 1988, p. 74)
3. *Theorem of Social Responsibility.* We must recognize (and make explicit) the potential and real harm of inadequate "family sociology" (as any other inadequate sociology) and, as a consequence, assert the importance

of developing a methodologically unified NEW "Family Studies" both to protect society and to benefit society. (Bernardes, 1988, p. 76)

The development of new and exciting approaches to "Family Studies" will yield a large range of highly valuable knowledge about "family life" that will enable us to more effectively deal with the whole range of social problems (Bernardes, 1997).

REFERENCES

Anderson, D. & Dawson, G. (1986). *Family portraits*. London: Social Affairs Unit.

Askham, J. (1984). *Identity and stability in marriage*. Cambridge: Cambridge University Press.

Backett, K. C. (1982). *Mothers and fathers: A study of the development and negotiation of parental behaviour*. London: Macmillan.

Ball, D. W. (1972). The "Family" as a sociological problem: Conceptualization of the taken-for-granted as prologue to social problems analysis. *Social Problems, 19* (3), 295-307.

Ball, D. W. (1975). Privacy, publicity, deviance and control. *Pacific Sociological Review, 18*(3), 259-278.

Barrett, M. (1980). *Women's oppression today: Problems of Marxist feminist analysis*. London: Verso.

Barrett, M., & McIntosh, M. (1991). *The anti-social family (Rev. ed.)*. London: Verso.

Beechey, V. (1985). Familial ideology. In V. Beechey & J. Donald (Eds.), *Subjectivity and social relations* (pp. 98-120). Open University Press, Milton Keynes.

Bender, D. R. (1967). A refinement of the concept of household: Families, co-residence and domestic functions. *American Anthropologist, 69* (6), 493-504.

Berger, P. L., Kellner, H. (1971). Marriage and the construction of reality: An exercise in the microsociology of knowledge. In B. R. Cosin (Ed.), *School and society: A sociological reader* (pp. 23-31). London: Routledge Kegan Paul & Open University Press.

Bernardes, J. (1985a). Do we really know what the family is? In P. Close & R. Collins (Eds.), *Family and economy in modern society* (pp. 192-211). Basingstoke: Macmillan.

Bernardes, J. (1985b). "Family Ideology": Identification and exploration. *Sociological Review, 33* (2), 275-297.

Bernardes, J. (1986a). Multidimensional developmental pathways: A proposal to facilitate the conceptualisation of "family diversity." *Sociological Review, 34* (3), 590-610.

Bernardes, J. (1986b). Research note: In search of "The Family": Analysis of the 1981 United Kingdom census. *Sociological Review, 34* (4), 828-836.

Bernardes, J. (1987). Doing things with words: Sociology and "family policy" debates. *Sociological Review, 35* (3), 679-702.

Bernardes, J. (1988). Founding the new "Family Studies." *Sociological Review, 36* (1), 57-86.

Bernardes, J. (1991). *The development of a family policy programme in Europe: A report.* Paper presented to the Second Annual European Research Conference, University of Nottingham.

Bernardes, J. (1995). *Family organisations and associations in the United Kingdom: A directory.* London: Family Policy Studies Centre.

Bernardes, J. (1997). *Family studies: An introduction.* London: Routledge.

Bjornberg, U. (1992). *Parenting in transition.* In U. Bjornberg (Ed.), European parents in the 1990s: Contradictions and comparisons (pp. 1-41). London: Transaction.

Bowley, A. L., & Hogg, M. H. (1925). *Has poverty diminished?* London: King and Son.

Brannen, J., & Wilson, G. (1987). *Give and take in families: Studies in resource distribution.* London: Allen and Unwin.

Buck, N., & Scott, J. (1994). Household and family change. In N. Buck et al., (Eds.), *Changing households: The British household panel survey 1990-1992* (pp. 61-82). University of Essex: ESRC Centre on Micro-Social Change.

Burr, W. R. et al. (1988). Epistemologies that lead to primary explanations in family science. *Family Science Review, 1* (3), 185-210.

Cheal, D. (1991). *Family and the state of theory.* Harvester, NY: Wheatsheaf.

Cohen, G. (1987). Introduction: The economy, the family, and the life course. In G. Cohen (Ed.), *Social Change and the Life Course* (pp 1-32). London: Tavistock.

Collier, J. et al (1982). Is there a family? New anthropological views. In B. Thorne & M. Yalom (Eds.), *Rethinking the Family* (pp. 245-58). NY: Longman.

DeVault, M. L. (1991). *Feeding the family: The social organization of caring as gendered work.* Chicago: University of Chicago Press.

Doherty, W. J., & Campbell, T. L. (1988). *Families and health.* Beverly Hills, CA: Sage.

Donati, P. (1991). The development of European policies for the protection of families and children: Problems and prospects. Paper presented at the EC conference on child, family, and society, Luxembourg.

Durham, M. (1985). Family, morality and the new right. *Parliamentary Affairs, 38* (2), 180-91.

Feminist Review. (1988). Family secrets: Child sexual abuse. *Special Edition*, No. 28.

Finch, J. (1989). *Family obligations and social change.* Cambridge: Polity.

Fitzgerald, T. (1983). The new right and the family. In M. Loney et al. (Eds), *Social Policy and Social Welfare* (pp. 46-58). Open University Press, Milton Keynes.

Gershuny, J. et al. (1994). Introducing household panels. In N. Buck et al., *Changing Households* (pp. 10-26). University of Essex: ESRC Centre on Micro-Social Change.

Gubrium, J. F., & Holstein, J. A. (1990). *What Is family?* Mountain View, CA: Mayfield.

Gubrium, J. F., & Lynott, R. J. (1985). Family rhetoric as social order. *Journal of Family Issues, 6* (1), 129-152.

Levin, I. (1990). How to define family. *Family Reports, 17.* Uppsala: Uppsala Universitet.

Mannheim, K. (1972). *Ideology and utopia: An introduction to the sociology of knowledge*. London: Routledge & Kegan Paul.

Mayer, J. E. (1967a). People's imagery of other families. *Family Process, 6* (1), 27-36.

Mayer, J. E. (1967b). The invisibility of married life. *New Society, 230* (23 February), 272-273.

Morgan, D. H. M. (1985). *The family, politics and social theory*. London: Routledge & Kegan Paul.

Murphy, M. (1983). The life course of individuals in the family: Describing static and dynamic aspects of contemporary family. In British Society for Population Studies, *The family* (pp. 50-70). London: OPCS.

Nunnally, E. W. (1988). Troubled relationships. In C. S. Chilman, F. M. Cox & E. W. Nunally (Eds.), *Families in trouble series* (Vol. 30). Newbury Park: Sage.

Oakley, A. (1974). *The sociology of housework*. London: Martin Robertson.

Oakley, A. (1981). *From here to maternity*. Harmondsworth: Penguin.

Oakley, A. (1982a). Conventional families. In R. Rapoport et al., *Families in Britain* (pp. 123-137). London: Routledge & Kegan Paul.

Oakley, A. (1982b). *Subject women*. New York: Pantheon Books.

Office of Population Censuses and Surveys (OPCS). (1992a). *Census 1991-Household Composition*. London: HMSO.

(Office of Population Censuses and Surveys (OPCS). (1992b). *General Household Survey-1991*. London: HMSO.

Ramey, J. (1978). Experimental family forms: The family of the future. *Marriage & Family Review, 1* (1), 1-9.

Rapoport, R., & Rapoport, R. N. (1977). *Mothers and others*. London: Routledge & Kegan Paul.

Rapoport, R., & Rapoport, R. N. (1982). *Families in Britain*. London: Routledge & Kegan Paul.

Ribbens, J. (1994). *Mothers and their children: A feminist sociology of childrearing*. London: Sage.

Ricketts, W., & Achtenberg, R. (1989). Adoption and foster parenting for lesbians and gay men: Creating new traditions in family. *Marriage & Family Review, 14* (3/4), 83-118.

Rimmer, L., & Wicks, M. (1981). The family today. *MOST-Journal of Modern Studies Association, 27* (Autumn), 1-4.

Rossi, A. (1977). A biosocial perspective on parenting. *Daedalus, 106* (2), 1-31.

Segal, L. (1983). *What is to be done about the family?* Harmondsworth: Penguin.

Shipman, M. D. (1981). *The limitations of social research (Rev. ed.)*. Harlow, Essex: Longman.

Stacey, J. (1990). *Brave new families: Stories of domestic upheaval in late twentieth century America*. NY: Basic.

Sussman, M. B. (1973). Non-traditional family forms in the 1970s. Minneapolis, MN: National Council on Family Relations.

Sussman, M. B. (1975). The second experience: Variant family forms. Minneapolis, MN: National Council on Family Relations.

Trost, J. (1988). Conceptualising the family. *International Sociology, 3*, 301-308.

Trost, J. (1990). Do we mean the same by the concept of family? *Communication Research, 17*(4), 431-43.

Weeks, J. (1986). *Family studies: Information needs and resources.* Yorkshire: British Library.

Westwood, S. (1984). *All day every day: Factory and family in the making of women's lives.* London: Pluto.

Whitfield, R. (1987). *Families matter.* London: Marshall Pickering.

Wilson, E. O. (1975). *Sociobiology: The new synthesis.* Cambridge, MA: Harvard University Press.

Zinn, M. B., & Eitzen, D. S. (1990). *Diversity in families.* NY: Harper and Row.

The Family in Jewish Tradition

Shlomo A. Sharlin

INTRODUCTION

The family is a feature of human society that predates modern thinking about it. Although the precise origin of the family is unknown, there is evidence of family life in every record of early mankind. It is found in every known society, both civilized and preliterate. An accurate sociological description of the family and its legal status in Biblical times is not readily available, as the relevant evidence is not of a strictly socio-descriptive nature.

The lack of suitable documents dealing with everyday life makes it necessary to utilize literary allusions in developing a picture of the family and its functions in Biblical times. The use of these literary images as a basis for framing a discussion of family in many eras and historical transitions suggests that a shared knowledge of what was noted could help unwind some of the assumptions that define family in terms of sociological discourse. The Book of Genesis, which contains stories of the patriarchs and their families, is the original source for forming images and deriving values of Jewish family life in the classical tradition. One focal point for tales of family life is the period of occupation and settlement in the land of Canaan. A second source of information is genealogies, found particularly in Genesis and in Chronicles, which depict the family trees of the main tribal leaders and groups.

Strictly legal passages in the Bible on the subject of family law are few in number, scattered throughout, and of limited scope. Social legislation pertaining specifically to the family is found primarily in Deuteronomy, including the laws relating to Levirate marriage (Deut. 25:5-10) and a brief outline of the process of divorce (Deut. 24:1-4). Although discoveries from ancient

Shlomo A. Sharlin is Director, Center for Research & Study of the Family, School of Social Work, University of Haifa, Haifa 31 999, Israel.

[Haworth co-indexing entry note]: "The Family in Jewish Tradition." Sharlin, Shlomo A. Co-published simultaneously in *Marriage & Family Review* (The Haworth Press, Inc.) Vol. 28, No. 3/4, 1999, pp. 43-54; and: *Concepts and Definitions of Family for the 21st Century* (ed: Barbara H. Settles et al.) The Haworth Press, Inc., 1999, pp. 43-54. Single or multiple copies of this article are available for a fee from The Haworth Document Delivery Service [1-800-342-9678, 9:00 a.m. - 5:00 p.m. (EST). E-mail address: getinfo@haworthpressinc.com].

Israel have not yielded any legal documents pertaining to marriage, it is believed that such documents were used by the Israelites in matters of marriage and divorce. Written marriage contracts are not mentioned until a later period. As a result of such limited sources, therefore, no early Jewish writing was devoted specifically to the family, and no straightforward definition of the family can be found in the Bible or other early sacred writings. The Talmud, encompassing the written laws governing all aspects of life, devoted a whole book to marriage and to divorce, but none to the functions of the family. Most of what we know about the family was established during the period of the Bible, and very little has been added until modern times.

MARRIAGE, PROCREATION, AND DIVORCE

Leviticus gives the "forbidden degrees," that is, a list of those relationships that were considered consanguineous (blood relations or 'near kin') and, therefore, made marriage forbidden. The Bible strictly prohibited marriage among consanguineous relatives, and the ties of blood relationship that forbade sexual relations were spelled out in order to prevent any violations (Lev. 18:6-18; 20:11-14; 17:19-21). These taboos included 26 relationships considered as "secondary incest," such as daughter-in-law or sister-in-law. No restrictions were placed, however, on marrying within the extended family; instead these marriages were accepted and even encouraged.

The Israelite family as reflected in all genealogical and narrative sources was patriarchal. There is no word in the Old Testament that corresponds precisely to the modern "nuclear family," consisting of father, mother and children. The closest equivalent to the family in the Bible was aptly termed "bet av" or "father's house" (Gen. 24:38), with the establishment of a new family being termed "house building" (Deut. 25:10). This household, composed of several generations, was formed by parents, children, sons- and daughters-in-law, as well as dependents. The father was the head of the Biblical family unit, the owner of family property, and the person through whom genealogy was traced.

The family (father's house) was tied through various relationships to a much broader circle of family relatives that included the parents' brothers, particularly from the father's side, their in-laws and their children. The term "bayit" or "house" usually described a subdivision of the "mishpahah" (which refers to the "clan" or "family" in the larger sense) (Josh. 7:14) and the "shevet" (or "tribe") (Ex. 12:21). Even the nation ("am") or the "house of Israel" was considered to be an extension of the family (Num. 25:15). In fact, the root of the word "mishpahah" means to incorporate or to bind together, and, as such, the concept of family was rather loosely defined.

The concept of the family, therefore, included numerous "father-houses" and the resulting kinship of all the persons constituting such a political division. This division held from generation to generation and was usually named after an ancient father who was a common ancestor. Thus, family was viewed not only as a smaller, nuclear unit, but also as an extended framework for a larger unit of society. The criteria for membership in a family (in the broader sense) were blood relationship and descent from a common ancestor; legal ties, such as common habitation and marriage; and geographical proximity.

The genealogies of I Chronicles sometimes refer to the clan leader as the "father" of a town or towns in his district (I Chron. 2:51-52). A common livelihood or profession was probably a major factor in family and clan solidarity. Besides those families who engaged primarily in farming their own lands, there were others who practiced a specific trade. From an economic standpoint, the larger family was the strongest and most stable institution, while the smaller "father-houses" were split and eventually disappeared.

Roles and Functions in the Family

As a social institution, the family provided a framework for regulating sexual relations, conserving lines of descent, securing property ownership, dictating inheritance rights, and executing justice. It also assigned roles for the division of labor and the responsibility for socializing children, as well as defining the roles of its members in relation to the external world. In the Bible, the division between the roles of women and men in daily family life was sharply drawn. The men were dominant in the public sphere, as leaders in the political arena, while the women dominated the private sphere, confining themselves to domestic duties such as cooking.

The head of the Biblical family was the patriarch who exercised authority over his wife and children (Num. 26:54-55). Marriage was based primarily on the patriarchal model with the woman joining and enlarging her husband's family, and virtually becoming his possession (Ex. 20:14). A woman was required to go along with her husband into servitude if he could not repay his debts (Ex. 21:2-3); however, she was not a slave that he might sell as he could his daughter.

Despite subordination to their husbands, women retained some rights, such as possessing and trading property even while married, and inheriting property from their fathers in the absence of sons (Num. 26:28-34; 27:1-11). At the death of a husband, a woman could become the actual, and probably the legal, head of the household if there were no sons of responsible age (II Kings 8:1-6).

Women were not simply portrayed as docile characters who were subservient to their husbands' authority. They argued (Gen. 30:1) and gave orders

(Gen. 16:2); some had very strong characters, even if their power was not always displayed openly. The influence of famous mothers in epic tradition, such as Sarah (Gen. 21:12), is illustrative of the significance attached to their role. While the status of the woman in the family was not nearly as high as her husband's, she was considered to be the undisputed mistress of the household. In bearing sons, she gave to the tribe its most valuable possession, and as such, her position did afford her some compensations.

The modern definitions of monogamy and polygamy were not strictly applicable to the ancient world. Polygamy was commonly practiced by men who held two or more wives at a time. However, a woman had an advantage if she were the senior wife of a harem or the sole wife of a monogamous marriage. Wives had their own private rooms that no strange man was allowed to enter; yet, they were by no means forbidden to associate with men and even took part at banquets.

Despite the practice of polygamy, the taboo against adultery was enforced as one of the Ten Commandments, and violations were severely punished. The law operated on a double standard and was much stricter for women, whose infidelity was punishable with death by stoning. The adulterer was not punished unless he committed the crime with a married woman. In that case, his sin was considered to be a violation of the husband's rights, while the adulteress was viewed as a wicked woman responsible for wounding the honor of her husband and destroying the basis of the family (Num. 5:11-31).

The most important function of the wife was the bearing of children. In accordance with the command to "be fruitful and multiply" (Gen. 1:28), procreation was regarded as the supreme duty. Motherhood was considered a blessing, and childlessness the greatest misfortune, even a punishment from God (Gen. 30:23). The number of children a woman had influenced her status, whereas her honor deteriorated within the family if she proved unable to bear children. As a mother, particularly of a son, a woman occupied a position of distinction within the family. Sons were especially desired because they alone assured the continuity of the family name, and the absence of sons threatened a man's house with extinction (Num. 27:4,8). Without sons, a man perceived himself as a "dried up wood" because after his death, his name would be forgotten (Gen. 29:30-31). The father's first-born son held a special position above his brothers and was entitled to double inheritance over them (Deut. 21:15-17).

If a woman was barren, her husband was entitled to take either another wife or a concubine. According to Jewish law, servants were considered to be part of the family (Gen. 12:16). In fact, the word "servant" shares the same root with the word "family." Thus, the wife might voluntarily offer her handmaiden for childbearing purposes in order to protect her status as well as to ensure the inheritance of her home (Gen. 16:1-2). The legal status of the concubine was lower than that of the wife, and her children were not necessarily entitled to inherit equally. Biblical law insisted, however, that they should not be completely deprived of their rights (Gen. 21:10; 25:6).

The distinction between legitimacy and illegitimacy in their present significance did not exist. Insofar as the father was known, all children were considered to be legitimate, whether borne by concubines or lawful wives (Gen. 21:10). The subject of adoption, as used today in its legal meaning, is not mentioned directly in the Bible; nevertheless, some clues can be found that it was practiced. Adoption was not addressed as such probably due to the great importance attached to family boundaries and the significance of blood relations within the social organization.

Divorce

Childlessness was the most common motive for a man to divorce his wife. So essential was procreation as a purpose of marriage that a man was not only permitted, but even encouraged, to divorce his wife after ten years of barrenness (Yev. 6:6). According to Biblical law, it was only the husband who was allowed to take the initiative in a divorce proceeding and could do so with or without the consent of his wife (Deut. 24:1-4). This did not change until the turn of the 11th century, when Gershom ben Judah ruled that a divorce could be implemented only with the consent of both parties.

Although divorce was permitted in the Bible and the Talmud, overall it was frowned upon by the sages. Despite this reluctance, however, the sages did lay down the grounds for divorce by both the husband and the wife (Git. 90a). In practice, divorce was a rarity in Jewish communities and was considered a stigma. The powerful bond which united parents and children with mutual responsibilities was expected to strengthen the family unit enough to enable it to withstand all stresses, both internal and external.

THE ESSENCE OF FAMILY LIFE

Domestic harmony was an ideal toward which Jewish families strove. The guidelines for achieving this harmony were clearly outlined: "A man should spend less than his means on food, up to his means on clothes, and beyond his means in honoring wife and children because they are dependent on him" (Hul. 84b). Yet, harmony was achieved not only through the give and take of interpersonal relationships, but also through the experience of ritual and holy events. The customs and strong values inherent in the Jewish way of life served to unify the family and sustain family bonds even in the hardest of times.

There was great emphasis placed on the value of the family as the social unit responsible for nurturing domestic and religious virtues. This resulted in the Jewish home becoming the most vital factor in the survival of Judaism and the preservation of the Jewish way of life, more so even than the synagogue or school in later times. The traditional Jewish home was the center of religious practice and ceremony, with a religious spirit of observance dictating dietary habits and other aspects of daily life.

The family unit was regarded somewhat as a closed one (Num. 24:5). Usually a woman and her children would reside in her own tent or house, thereby forming sub-groups of mothers' children (Gen. 30:14-16). Within these units, the first-born male would instruct and protect his brothers. By subdividing the family into small units centered around the mother, women were able to enjoy rights and roles that the written law did not allow. Thus, a woman could function as a ruler in her own domicile, even if not on a legal basis.

The mother was primarily responsible for the early training and education of her children (Prov. 1:8) until they grew older (6 years old) and the father assumed his duties of teaching his children religion, Jewish values, and moral behavior (Gen. 18:19, Ex. 12:26-27). It was the father's duty to teach his sons a craft or trade, while mothers taught their daughters at home about the domestic responsibilities of a Jewish woman. Special weight was laid upon early religious training, as the family functions were religious as well as social.

The wealthier class also used special tutors to teach reading and writing. There is, however, no mention of school in the Old Testament. Schools were established at a much later period, and then only in the larger cities. Education was always considered to be important, and all knowledge was based on fear of God and obedience to parents (Prov. 1:7).

Children were expected to "honor" and "revere" both parents and to demonstrate their respect through obedience (Ex. 20:12, Deut. 21:18-21). This commandment required that children refrain from sitting in their parents' seats (a practice that is followed even in modern times), interrupting them, or taking sides in a dispute. Strict discipline was maintained, and children who assaulted or even cursed their parents could be punished by the death penalty (Ex. 21:15-17); a rebellious son was to be stoned to death (Deut. 21:18-21). According to the Talmud, this practice was never enacted, though the threat served as a deterrent to rebellious behavior.

As the head of the family, the father's authority over his children was almost absolute. Children were regarded as the father's property and could be seized for payment of debt (II Kings 4:1). His control included the right to sell a daughter into marriage, although there were limitations on selling her into slavery (he could not sell her to foreigners). Moreover, an absolute ban existed on selling daughters into prostitution (Ex. 21: 7-11, Lev. 19:29).

Historically, children were viewed as extensions of their parents and were pressured to conform to their expectations. A son was expected to grow up into a scholar, and likewise to bring honor to the family by marrying the daughter of a scholar. Genealogical lists were drawn up and carefully preserved to monitor the purity of the family. The status of certain families as "pure" and "impure" was well known, and references were made to "families of scribes which produced scribes, of scholars who produced scholars, and of plutocrats who produced plutocrats" (Eccl. R. 4:9).

Both purity of descent and health considerations were regarded as important, and there were warnings against marrying into a family with a history of such diseases as epilepsy or leprosy (Yev. 64b). By custom, marriages outside the clan were discouraged, while marriages with relations within the extended family were preferred. Because marriage was a question of admitting a woman into the family, it became a family affair. Consequently, it was greatly frowned upon for the son to marry a woman against the will of his parents.

The responsibility of the individual member of a family towards the good name of the family as a whole is constantly stressed. This is evident from the many Biblical passages delivering the message:

> A family is like a heap of stones. Remove one, and the whole structure can collapse. (Gen. R. 100:7)
> Whosoever brings disrepute upon himself brings disrepute upon his whole family. (Num. R. 21:3)

Here too, the family is perceived as a "system" to which modern system concepts apply. This strong regard for the family honor gave rise to the ceremony of "kezazah" in which all the members of the family participated when one of them married a woman who was not considered to be worthy of them (Ket. 28b). Such heavy emphasis on the worthiness of the family as a prime consideration in choosing a marriage partner has persisted throughout the history of Jewish social life. This is symbolically reflected in the notion that still exists today that one should be able to "sit down at the table" with the respective families of the potential bride and groom.

Family honor was also used as the basis for justifying the system of retribution. Family solidarity was demonstrated through customs such as blood revenge that was exacted upon members of another clan who had killed a kinsman. A whole family could be held responsible for one member's wrongdoing on the premise that

> there is not a family containing a publican of which all the members are not publicans or containing a thief in which they are not all thieves. (Shev. 39a)

Members of the same family were perceived as "brothers," and the relationship between brothers was highly significant in the Israelite family. Blood revenge was the primary responsibility of the immediate family relatives of the victim (Num. 35:9-34; Deut. 19:1-13). However, in the absence of a brother or another close relative, the circle of people who were responsible for the revenge was enlarged. The extended family then had to select the avenger (go'el) who would be considered as a "brother."

Thus, each member of the group was entitled to protection by that group, and the avenger had obligations extending to many matters of family honor. When brothers departed from each other in order to establish a new "father-house" of their own, they were still tied to each other with a reciprocal responsibility to protect and support each other. A near kinsman was required to redeem a relative who had been forced by poverty to sell his land or other family property or to sell himself into slavery to pay a debt (Lev. 25:25, 47-49).

It was even the responsibility of a man to marry his brother's widow if he died without sons to take over the household. This was the practice of the Levirate marriage that was instituted to carry on the name of the deceased brother and to ensure the continuance of his estate. Thus, the son born of such a marriage was considered as the child of the deceased (Deut. 25: 5-10). Later, daughters were given the right to inherit in the absence of sons, thereby enabling the preservation of the family estate. At that point, the Levirate requirements became limited to cases in which the deceased had left no children at all (Num. 27:4).

DISCUSSION

As evident from this discussion of the family in Jewish tradition, most of what the term "family" describes was established during the Biblical period and remained largely unchanged until the last century. Very little was added during the subsequent periods of the Settlement, the Kingdom, and the Second Temple until modern times.

Most major family concepts, such as family structure, mate selection, engagement, marriage, inheritance and divorce, including adultery and incest, were all established during the Biblical period. No recorded changes are known during the Settlement and Kingdom periods. The controversy between monogamy and polygamy continues as a result of influence by other nations. Very few changes took place during the Babylonian period (after the destruction of the Second Temple). The dowry was replaced by the marriage contract ("Ktuba"), and the engagement and marriage ceremonies were combined into one. Whereas the age of marriage during Biblical times was "when the children grow up," namely, 12 for girls and 13 for boys, it rose to

18 during the Mishna and Talmud period (4th Century). At that time, the marriage certificate became an official contract, thus protecting the woman against a forced divorce. No major changes or additions were found during the Middle Ages, with the exception of Rabbi Gershon's improvement in the 11th Century. This principle stipulated that a man could not marry two women, nor divorce his wife against her will. An exception occurred only if the wife was mentally ill, a circumstance meaning that a second wife could be taken. Capital punishment and killing for blood revenge, of course, have long since been abolished.

The subject of the family during Biblical times must be regarded, therefore, under two aspects: one, the family in its wider sense of individuals related by marriage or common ancestry; and two, the smaller family unit consisting of parents and children. In Jewish tradition, the family constitutes a very closely knit unit in which all members are bound by mutual ties of responsibility. These ties provided the primary focus of Biblical life, and considerable attention was given to the interactions of various family members within the context of the patriarchal community. Biblical heroes did not attain identity and glory away from their families, and their problems and preoccupations were deeply domestic. Because family was the point around which life revolved, it was simultaneously the source of intimate connection and the scene of spiritual struggle.

In the post-Biblical period, as the land was settled and interaction with institutions outside the structure of the family developed, the ties of the larger clan tended to weaken and the smaller monogamous family unit took on increasing importance. Although polygamy was permitted by both the Bible and the Talmud, the ideal set forth was always of husband, wife, and children forming one unit. The passage from Psalms, "thy wife shall be a fruitful vine in the innermost part of thy house; thy children like olive plants round about thy table" (Ps. 128:2-3), formed the basis of innumerable homilies in the Talmud extolling the virtues of domestic bliss. Finally in the year 1000, monogamy was formally decreed as the normal state of marriage by Gershom ben Judah.

The pattern of Jewish family life set down in the Talmud was the model and practice until modern times. The age of marriage was set at 18 (Avot. 5:24), although some sages encouraged earlier marriage (Kid. 29b). Marriages were usually arranged by the parents of both families, with the betrothal being considered a formal marriage that could be dissolved only through divorce or death. Sexual life was strictly regulated and great importance was attached to ritual aspects; celibacy was discouraged and rare. The Talmud pointed to the Biblical verse, "he created it (the world) not a waste; he formed it to be inhabited" (Is. 45:18), as a justification for the religious duty not only to marry but also to establish a family.

CONCLUSION

The family was regarded as the smallest social unit through which the cultural and religious heritage of Judaism could be transmitted. The sanctity of the home was especially apparent in Jewish life during the Middle Ages. Throughout those centuries of persecution and migration, the home became the pillar of moral and social strength and the key to maintaining a Jewish consciousness. The observances of the faith were so entwined with the daily customs of the home that Jewish religion and its family life became bonded as one.

The Jewish tradition did not distinguish between religious rules, moral behavior, and law, but demanded that all be equally followed by the people. Those persons who did not perform accordingly would be bound by social sanctions. Such orders were based on God's commandments rather than on logical constructs. Throughout the coming centuries, even while the law evolved into a different form of government executed by court houses, this set of orders remained in force only on the basis of social sanctions.

Thus, in the beginning, Biblical law took the form of religious charisma that was maintained as God's law, and only much later was the legal process assumed by the "dayanim" (religious judges). Since Jewish tradition is based on the Halacha (Jewish law), it does not recognize a Jewish nation that is not a Biblical nation.

Traditional practices were maintained and reinforced within the context of the Jewish family, whose concepts and laws were as old as Biblical times. Consequently, the family served as a source of values and philosophy of life. Jewish values and Jewish traditions were transmitted from generation to generation within the family context. It is only in the last 200 years that this solid structure has begun to waver.

Jewish law has never lost its original character; but exists side by side with the State and even binds the State. In fact, the 1953 law of the Rabbinical Court (Marriage and Divorce) states clearly that all Jews residing in Israel as Israeli citizens will be under the jurisdiction of the Rabbinical law.

Despite the influence of tradition, the reality of the Jewish people since the 19th century has changed, and many Jews no longer live "by the Bible." Major changes in the status of women and the family have had a radical impact on modern society. Social and demographic trends in Western society have brought changes in marriage and family life that have altered the family structure. The State of Israel has developed new laws in recent years to keep up with the changes created by the new era; these may not be sufficient and many more should follow.

Nevertheless, it is interesting to note that so many basic structures and functions of the family have never been changed or challenged. New laws can continue to be established without losing the ancient meanings and values. The old concepts can still be used; it is necessary only to adopt new laws and new sanctions rather than to replace the concepts themselves. For example, the stigma attached to adultery still exists even though it is no longer punished by public stoning. Another concept that is still alive is the familial responsibility to educate children, even though the specific parental roles spelled out in the Bible are no longer applicable to modern times.

All of the meanings that we attach to the structure and functions of the Jewish family were established very early in the history of Jewish social life. In this tradition, most of what the term "family" describes has been stable until the last century. Not only within the Jewish communities, but also in the general western secular society the concepts associated with the Biblical views of marriage, children, and family responsibilities are often retained in evaluating and interpreting social practice. However, it is useful to remember that these ideas are seen through the lens of contemporary problems and practice. This brief review of the major ideas in Jewish tradition of Biblical interpretation can be used to enlighten current debates on the family in today's policy work.

Despite the fact that there is not a current definition of the family that is universally accepted, the loosely defined family unit that is bound and incorporated together fits family systems theories and can be used for research in the social sciences. Even in the absence of a clear definition, however, we can continue to adapt the concept of family in our struggle to understand it. This process might help us account for the survival of the oldest institution on earth.

SELECTED SOURCES FOR ADDITIONAL INFORMATION

Biblical encyclopedia. (1968). (pp. 582-588). Jerusalem: Bialik.

Childress, J. F., & Macquarrie, J. (Eds.). (1986). *The Westminster dictionary of Christian ethics* (pp. 224-226). Philadelphia: The Westminster Press.

Cornfeld, G., & Luria, B. Z. (Eds). (1967). *Encyclopedia of the Bible and second temple* (Vol. 1, pp. 782-790; Vol. 2, pp. 408-418). Tel Aviv: Achiasaf.

Douglas, J. D. (Ed.). (1972). *The new Bible dictionary* (pp. 415-418). London: Inter-Varsity Press.

Encyclopedia Judaica. (1971). (Vol. 6, pp. 1164-1172). Jerusalem: Keter House, Ltd..

Ferm, V. (Ed.). (1964). *An encyclopedia of religion* (pp. 271-272). Paterson, New Jersey: Littlefield, Adams & Co.

Harley, D. (1982). *The world's religions.* Tel Aviv: Devir Publishing.

Hoffman, Y. (Ed). (1988). *The Israeli encyclopedia of the Bible* (pp. 562-564). Massada.

Jackson, S. M. (Ed). (1967). *The new Schaff-Herzog encyclopedia of religious Knowledge* (pp. 273-277). Grand Rapids, Michigan: Baker Book House.

Lor, G. (1982). *The relationship between God and nation as man-woman relationship.* Unpublished dissertation (Chapter 1). The University of Haifa.

MacGregor, G. (1990). *The everyman dictionary of religion and philosophy* (pp. 191-192, 400). London: J. M. Dent & Sons, Ltd.

McGraw-Hill encyclopedia of world biography. (1973). (pp. 371-372).

Radi, Z. (1989). *The new Biblical dictionary.* (pp. 339-340).

Singer, I. (Ed). (1903). *The Jewish encyclopedia* (Vol. 5, pp. 337-338). New York and London: Funk and Wagnalls Company.

Solialy, M. (Ed). (1965). *Biblical lexicon* (pp. 576-581). Tel Aviv: Devir Publishing.

Wigoder, G. (Ed). (1989). *The encyclopedia of Judaism* (pp. 255-258, 284). NY: Macmillan Publishing Company.

APPENDIX

ABBREVIATIONS FOR BIBLICAL AND TALMUDIC SOURCES

Abbreviation	Source	Abbreviation	Source
Avot	Avot	Kid.	Kidushin
Chron. I, II	Chronicles	Kings I, II	Kings
Deut.	Deuteronomy	Hul.	Hulin
Eccl.	Ecclesiates	Lev.	Leviticus
Ex.	Exodus	Num.	Numbers
Gen.	Genesis	Prov.	Proverbs
Gen. R.	Genesis Raba	Ps.	Psalms
Git.	Gittin	Shev.	Shevuot
Is.	Isaiah	Yev.	Yevanot
Josh.	Joshua		

Redefining Western Families

John F. Peters

INTRODUCTION

Most adults reflect upon the past ten years and recognize change in their family. Those who are at least middle age generally recognize a lot of change, and the elderly even more change. For many, such contemplation produces thoughts of times when family was less complex and more connected or congenial. Coontz (1992) identifies this positive and often unreal reflection of family in the past as "nostalgia." This paper does not seek to evaluate whether our recollection of the past is correct or not. Rather, it seeks to identify significant areas of family change in contemporary society and to expand the definition of the family to more adequately fit the reality of today.

This paper does not attempt to be universal, comprehensive and inclusive of family over time and space. Historical and cross-cultural variations of family relate to such matters as marriage form (polygamy and polyandry), structures, kinship and socialization. This paper will address matters that relate to the definition of the family due to social and structural changes in the western world. Placing boundaries upon this broad subject of the definition of family makes this project manageable and realistic, as well as more pragmatic for research purposes.

The term "family" is one of the most misused concepts in the English language. It is more commonly used to refer to a group with biological ties with a minimum of two generations of people. More recently corporations,

John F. Peters is affiliated with the Department of Sociology and Anthropology, Wilfrid Laurier University, Waterloo, Ontario, Canada N2L 3C5.

This research was funded in part by a grant from Wilfrid Laurier University and is a revision of a paper presented at the International Sociological Association CFR Seminar in Norway, 1991.

[Haworth co-indexing entry note]: "Redefining Western Families." Peters, John F. Co-published simultaneously in *Marriage & Family Review* (The Haworth Press, Inc.) Vol. 28, No. 3/4, 1999, pp. 55-66; and: *Concepts and Definitions of Family for the 21st Century* (ed: Barbara H. Settles et al.) The Haworth Press, Inc., 1999, pp. 55-66. Single or multiple copies of this article are available for a fee from The Haworth Document Delivery Service [1-800-342-9678, 9:00 a.m. - 5:00 p.m. (EST). E-mail address: getinfo@haworthpressinc.com].

financial institutions, religious bodies, communes, and yacht clubs (Aversa, 1991) also use it to convey a loyal, caring and somewhat congenial collection of people with a degree of fraternity. In general, the term "family" carries a sense of the best in relationships. I now address several definitions used by academicians until about 1980.

CONVENTIONAL DEFINITIONS OF THE FAMILY

Murdock's (1949:1) definition of the family has been used for decades in both anthropology and sociology. He defines family as

> a social group characterized by common residence, economic coopera-tion, and reproduction. It includes adults of both sexes, at least two of whom maintain a socially approved sexual relationship, and one or more children, own or adopted, of the sexually cohabiting adults.

Coser (1964:xvi) has sought to be more precise, using a more functional definition. She states the family to be

> a group manifesting the following organizational attributes: It finds its origin in marriage; it consists of husband, wife, and children born in their wedlock, though other relatives may find their place close to this nuclear group, and the group is united by moral, legal, economic, religious and social rights and obligations (including sexual rights and prohibitions as well as such socially patterned feelings as love, attrac-tion, piety, and awe).

Stephens (1963:4) recognizes the family in the following way:

> a social arrangement based on marriage and the marriage contract, including recognition of the rights and duties of parenthood, common residence for husband, wife and children, and reciprocal economic obligations between husband and wife.

In the above definitions we find considerable similarity. Some common themes are economic cooperation, a heterosexual union of an adult male and female with recognized rights and obligations, children, and possibly a com-mon residence.

The traditional and more conventional usage of the nuclear family has reference to mother and father and their biological child(ren). It also em-braces widows and widowers and their children, as well as orphans who are adopted into a family. The term includes the remarriage of widow(er)s with or without children, even if one of the spouses is single. In the case of orphans, children are identified in the new family. But beyond these boundaries, the definition of the conventional family, until the seventies, has been limiting, even though other family-like configurations have existed.

The Problem of Definition in Contemporary Times

In the conventional sense we commonly distinguish between the extended and the nuclear family. We also make a difference between one's family of orientation and family of procreation. Even in the conventional sense it is conceivable to find oneself in several different families simultaneously without any problem linguistically, socially or even in terms of identity. To go beyond this more traditional grid of family often invites problems of definition in public usage. However, the more recent emphasis upon human rights and equality, the place of law in family, and feminism, force one to redefine family. What are the new boundaries for family?

With the general acceptance of separation and divorce in western societies after the mid-fifties the definition of family has expanded. The reconstituted household of one divorced adult bonded with another heterosexual adult with a custodial child or children is now generally accepted as family. Similarly we accept as family the household comprised of a single mother and her child(ren). Ultimately we ask what are the criterion of family? Is the definition dependent upon matters of residence, care, biology, history?

From the above expanded and more acceptable discussions of family definition we recognize several social groupings that require further consideration with attendant possibilities and problems. Which is the real family for the foster child: that of biology or residence? What of the cohabiting couple, when one adult has a child from a former relationship? And what of a widow and widower who remarry at age fifty-eight, and both have grown children who do not reside in the newly established household? Is family restricted to that of the married widow and widower? Are offspring in the previous marriages of these two included in the new family?

What of the woman who raises her granddaughter while the mother temporarily lives elsewhere? Does family include or exclude the child's non-custodial parent when the latter has infrequent or no contact with offspring? The term binuclear family (Ahrons, 1979) may be most appropriate for this situation. And, what about children who are wards of the state?

What of the gay couple in whose household there is a child from one of the adults' former heterosexual relationships? Are brother and sister who reside together family? Can two adults, either of the same or different sex who reside together be considered family? Or what of the non-related adult who resides in a family's household for many years and engages in virtually all family activities? And what of the same-sexed couple and children? The problem is somewhat alleviated if we allow for multiple family membership.

The answer is partially dependent upon the perspective of the person asked. The adopted child may recognize her family of orientation as the real family. The child's definition of family may differ along the family life cycle. Initially she may not recognize adopted "parents" as parents, but after a few years, with infrequent or no contact with her biological parents, she may feel comfortable with her adopted "parents" as parents. She may also be influenced by whether she has siblings, and whether they live in the same or another family of adoption. At the same time she may see herself as dutifully connected to two families: one biological and one social, economic and emotional. In brief, there are varying circumstances which alter one's family. The experience and the context are important. Identification with more than one family is realistic.

In recent decades the conventional definition of family has proven to be too simplistic and grossly inadequate. It has come under severe attack because of either excluding other family forms or holding one family type as superior to all others. Eichler (1990) recognizes that the family is not monolithic, and urged a more realistic expansion of the use of the term "family." She recognized family dimensions to be socialization, emotion, residence, economics, sexuality and reproduction. She posits that all these dimensions need not be present for the existence of family. Hofferth (1985) coined the term "benchmark family," because it was inferred to be a standard with all other family forms being inferior. Smith (1993) has the same general criticism and uses the label Standard North American Family or SNAF.

WHY A REDEFINITION OF THE FAMILY IS NECESSARY

I will address several reasons why the conventional definition of family is no longer satisfactory. First, many families are dysfunctional. Historically some families have always been dysfunctional, but currently the number and the complexity of family problems are overwhelming. Orthner (1995:15) notes that "there are not enough industry and government supports to compensate for many of the services that family members used to provide one another. . . . " No family agency or family researcher can realistically project a dramatic, significant, and positive change for this social problem. Some families appear to remain dysfunctional generation after generation.

Second, family needs to be redefined because family myths are being dispelled. Many of these myths have been constructed out of definitions of the benchmark or Standard North American Family. Until the sixties, activities of the family were considered private. With a few exceptions, the family was perceived as being good, stable and positive for each member. In more recent years we have become more public about real life within the family. Researchers have shown that family authority structures have been autocratic and patriarchal. Physical and mental violence in the family is pervasive. Even the elderly are sometimes abused by their very own adult children (Pillemer & Finkelhor, 1988; McDonald, Hornich, Robertson & Wallace, 1991; Larson, Goltz & Hobart, 1994).

Third, authority structures of the family are being radically changed (Peters, 1995). Women have participated in the work force outside the household in increasing numbers over the past fifty years, to the point that employment of both parents is normative. The current western lifestyle of consumerism dictates that the income of both parents is essential in almost all households. Married women's employment has raised their status and power in the household. Many partnerships in western families are no longer recognized as head-complement (e.g., husband/father as the dominant member and wife/mother as the subordinate member of a family), whereas only two generations earlier most partnerships were. Today the majority of western heterosexual relationships are junior-senior partners, and a few are equal partner relationships (Scanzoni, 1995). Some fathers are becoming more involved in child rearing. Men choose to be involved (Levy-Shiff & Israeliashvili, 1988; C. P. Cowan & P. A. Cowan, 1987; Larson, Goltz & Hobart, 1994).

Fourth, family experience has changed. Most westerners live in a very pluralistic society where children and parents are exposed to a range of family forms. Styles of family living vary by subculture, class, ethnicity, religion, region and generation. Television projects a plethora of family interaction, from the severe, sublime and abhorrent, to the humorous and ridiculous. Family values of morality are being challenged by other institutions. Children have a much greater age-graded experience that is reinforced in public school systems. Age cohorts experience their own culture of fads, fashions, language, acceptable behaviour and activity. Consumerism caters to this age grading of society.

Fifth, society's changing perceptions of gender require us to look more closely to definitions of family. All members of the family do not necessarily experience the same social class or social benefits. Husbands may live a life style that is superior to that of wives and children. This is further reinforced by many persons in the corporate world who live a life style at work that contrasts sharply to that of their own families. Feminists indelibly show that women have been and are in a subordinate status not only in the family, but in virtually all areas of society. This bifurcated system is viewed as unjustifiable and intolerable, and every effort is being made by feminists to rebuild our society to be liberated from gender inequality. This is a paradigm change. Most males and some females find this wave of change as inconvenient, unpredictable and even threatening. Many women and some men welcome the change, a radical modification for the traditional family. In the newer or wider family forms, roles are no longer determined by gender. Roles are determined by negotiation and choice, and can alter by circumstance, personal volition and normative changes in the family and life cycle (Marciano & Sussman, 1991).

Sixth, contact and interaction between adult males and females outside of the home environment are frequent, particularly at the place of work. Women are now co-workers in settings that were previously closed to them. Social and romantic exchanges may filter to the workplace as Scanzoni (1995:77) notes: "Close working relationships between women and men sometimes give rise to garbled sexual signals." These expanded working norms relating to gender relations have a different meaning for trust, fidelity and responsibility.

The seventh rationale for change in the definition of family is the legal dimension. In western societies the law has gargantuan implications upon the family. The law establishes an acceptable minimal age and in some cases a health examination for marriage. It dictates the conditions under which a marriage can be terminated, and the rights of each parent toward children after separation. The law can remove a child from a family deemed inappropriate for the child. Furthermore, in recent years the law has given children increasing rights, to the point where children have legally prosecuted parents. The government has and continues to play a pseudo-family or pro-family role in terms of financial aid: tax deductions, welfare, child bonus, unemployment moneys, pension and assistance for the handicapped or impaired. Pension moneys have been directed to the individual rather than the family unit, thus weakening the patriarchal structure, wherein mothers generally received moneys allocated for child care and housing.

The eighth reason why the conventional definition of family is inappropriate is the emphasis for civil and individual perceived rights over the rights or welfare of the collective. At times this countervails the best interest of the family. For example, the adult feels justified in terminating a relationship because it feels right, it is "where I'm at." In the youth culture, teenagers may ignore family prescriptions because of personal interests and goals. Family and group norms have definitely weakened. The immediate self-interest of the individual for divorce may have serious long-term consequences upon the family unit. Civil rights do not always place prime regard and respect upon the family. Furthermore, civil rights are universal rather than particular in nature. Codified legal rights may meet the needs of many, but do injustice in situations that are unique, or peculiar to a specific circumstance, time or subculture.

This individual characteristic of western cultures creates a definition of family by the individual. Thus, this definition is subjective, multiple, variable and changing. Theoretically the person at 22 may not identify parents and siblings as family because there is no co-residence, no financial exchange and no overt emotional bond. Similarly, teenagers may recognize peers as family above biological ties because of the time and quality of emotional exchange. The older person living alone may identify a pet dog as family.

TOWARDS A DEFINITION OF FAMILY

Over the past decade, the discussion over redefining the family has generated considerable heat. Bernardes (1986) argues that the term "family" is used so extensively, and with such a wide range of meaning, that it would be wise to drop the term altogether. In earlier and some more recent family research, discussion has centered upon family function. In the view of Collier, Rosaldo and Yanagisko (1982), such a perspective has given us an enormous broad scope as well as an expectation of good functioning families. They recognize that families are both nice and mean, patient and impatient, generous and miserly. Rather than to look at family as a concrete "thing" with concrete "needs," they advocate seeing the family as an ideological construct. At the same time, our ideology cannot exist in a state of limbo (Gittins, 1986). It has a relationship to people's actual behavior, or can at least be perceived as having such a relation. Such ideological attention might yield a more refined analysis of historical change in the Western family.

Marciano and Sussman (1991) simply used the term *wider families* in recognition of the significant family change in recent years. In the wider family there is not the limitation of age between children or even between partners, or even a recognition of siblings as seen in the conventional family. Children may precede rather than define the family. Legal marriage is not a binding force, because adult membership is a voluntary association. When relationships terminate, the division of property is made on the basis of law. Though kin bonds may be part of the wider family, these kinship bonds are incidental. Wider families show varying degrees of permanence and fluidity. There may be permanent severance, fragmentation, or reconstitution in a variety of forms. Wider families are autonomous, free and not coerced. Wider families become primary groups, making a "we" or an "in" group which contrasts with others and outsiders (Scanzoni & Marsiglio, 1995). The concept places emphasis upon openness and sensitivity rather than to a rigid definition or institution. This writer feels wider families must not be considered an alternative to family, but should be included in the usage of family in contemporary times.

Rapoport (1989) uses the *diversity model* in that the earlier family is pluralistic and has numerous alternatives. Cheal (1991) counters that such a term does not adequately identify the significant change in family and culture.

Stacey (1990:17) uses the term *postmodern family* "to signal the contested, ambivalent and undecided character of contemporary gender and kinship arrangements." She states that the modern family has given us chaos because of its structural fragility. The nature of the postmodern family is voluntary commitments by its members, showing itself as redefining, strengthening, weakening or abandonment. The postmodern family does not have the permanence or the optimism of the families found in the middle of this century (Cheal, 1993). Baudrillard (1983) concurs with this type of skepticism. The nature of the social is no longer one of unity and predictability, but of nodes of sociality within a constant flow of people, things and messages.

Gittins (1986) has probed the universality of the family and comes to three conclusions: Families must have some notion of co-residence; families have relationships and relationships are formed in a variety of ways; and relationships may be brief and are not necessarily natural. Furthermore, she feels the family is a strong symbol-system, and that it is necessary to 'deconstruct' many assumptions about the family.

One of the central notions of the contemporary family is nurturance. Scanzoni (1995) goes beyond nurturance, and sees the challenge of the contemporary family to be responsibility. His use of the term, responsibility, allows for much change and variation in bonding. Scanzoni (1995) says that we continually create a social family and therefore should redefine the concept to the reality of the present times and the current culture. He feels that family relationships are in flux, that this flux or change is normal in North American society, and that people adapt to these changing partnerships. This is evident in the more liberal acceptance and practice of premarital sex, the divorce rate and subsequent bonding of many couples, cohabitation and gay relationships. Bonding or "we-ness" is important in relationships (Scanzoni, 1995). Persons go through several different levels of bonding beginning with companionship, and then intimacy that may include sex. The next stage is the erotic relationship that includes the formation and maintenance phases, the latter involving sexual exclusivity. Even in the latter phase the individual is "available" to another bond should some set of circumstances threaten or terminate the existing couple-ness. Scanzoni's radical stance shifts the family focus away from the "until death do us part" promise (a permanent relationship ideal), or the restrictions of a legal marriage. He does not preclude that sexual fidelity is a basic criterion for adults in family. While he has done well in indicating that the redefining of family continually takes place within any culture, and particularly the changeability of adult unions, his focus is primarily that of coupling. He does not appreciate the degree to which bonds continue to exist primarily because of blood, which in many cases is "thicker than water." He overlooks the child factor.

ESTABLISHING CRITERIA FOR REDEFINING FAMILY

Any definition of family that restricts itself to two heterosexual adults is clearly inadequate. The question remains as to how far the boundaries of family can be stretched. People are in flux in their relationships, which have both social or legal implications. With the exception of the aged person without spouse, sibling, or offspring, virtually all persons have family ties in the traditional and biological sense. In reality all people have family-like ties: consisting, at a minimum, of bonds of emotion, economics or blood. These bonds understandably shift over time. Individuals may find themselves attached in some way to more than one family system. The family researcher will find it difficult to redefine family in a way that is acceptable to all people, or to all who take more than a miminal interest in family. Therefore the researcher is unlikely to find a universal definition to suit all scholars, let alone the public.

Self-Perception. The social scientist must be aware of at least four interpretations of family. The first of these is self-perception. Undoubtedly features that are perceived as closely related to family such as caring, loving, present in times of need, and long-term relationships might be fairly significant. The 15-year-old neighbor who "sleeps over" and goes to her friend's house frequently might be introduced as "one of the family." Two unrelated women who have lived together with no sexual relations, but with economic and emotional sharing, may consider themselves to be family. The person, irrespective of age, who has boarded or lived with a more conventional type of family for a long period of time might also be considered family. A few, and particularly elderly lone persons, may consider their pet as family. They share the same residence, there is an emotional bond, and the person often gives scrupulous care and time to the pet(s). The meaning of the relationship is significant to the individual. In each case there is long-term companionship, and in some cases co-residence. These relationships will have their own set of expectations and obligations.

Public Perception. The second interpretation of relevance to family definition is public perception. Public is defined in this article as a second person, a group, community, subculture or culture. Since humans are social beings, this interpretation affects one's personal definition of family, though it may not be identical to that held by the individual. There may be a difference between what *they* think and what *I* think, how *they* enact family and how *I* enact family. A child becomes aware of family definition variations when she/he finds that the neighbor's child gets paid for mowing the lawn or cleaning one's room, and he/she does not. The public has definitions of family that relate to sexual orientation of adults, duration and quality of the relationship, and the sharing of resources, space and time. Some would also include how the relationship was initiated, whether by priest, law or simply living together. Public perceptions of family vary by geography, age cohort, gender, social class, and religious affiliation. Public perceptions often stereotype some persons in families, stigmatize others, and in democratic societies have some direct or indirect bearing upon the third interpretation of the family.

Law. The third consideration of interpretation of family in western society is law. Law has an increasing impact upon the western families. Even though one of Canada's prime ministers stated that " . . . government has no business in a person's bedroom," the state appears to be omnipresent. The state has set the criterion of a legal will. The state has fixed the criterion by which property is divided between partners should a separation occur. The state has sought to establish a no-fault divorce process. More recently several countries have abolished any reference to bastard or illegitimate children. The state sets the rights and privileges of the non-custodial parent. The state has established the rights of the non-custodial father to his child born out of wedlock. The law has specific rules regarding the care of foster children or the adoption of children.

There are a number of current family issues which the law is in some way addressing (sometimes by neglect): abortion, child rights, parentage of surrogate children, life termination of the ill, visiting rights of next of kin for the hospital patient, homosexual marriages, benefits for gay and lesbian partners, family policy. These concerns of the general public are often addressed by specific regions (state or province) rather than on the federal level. We see considerable variation from one region to another. Therefore a universal definition of family would hardly be appropriate where legal factors play an important focus. At the same time we recognize that the law is not always consistent. For example, while the federal law may recognize a marriage, Canadian immigration authorities do not recognize a marriage of convenience (a marriage for the purpose of facilitating someone to enter Canada). The same applies for cohabitation. After three years of cohabiting, one is in many ways legally recognized as married. However, for their purposes, Canadian Immigration is not prepared to accept this legal definition.

History and Tradition. The fourth consideration of redefining the family is history and tradition. One must at the very least recognize the definition of family as used in recent history. This involves expectations and practices relating to law, religion, ethnicity, social groups and intra-family relationships. These historic usages have implications upon current definitions. (Studies in the history of family will undoubtedly expose irregularities and inconsistencies in commonly held views of the historical family.)

The family researcher will apply the methods of science that have been established and used over the past century. The researcher's investigation into family, though loaded with potential bias, is subject to the same vigor and scrutiny of any other science. We may have to resign ourselves to living with the ambivalence found in defining family. We have no difficulty in researching such social phenomenon as group, institution and community, all of which show a wide range of meaning to both the public and the researcher. The same applies to the concept of family.

Family researchers are accustomed to differentiating families: single parents, stepparenting, teenage motherhood, lesbian couples, the sandwiched generation. Such a focus has enriched our understanding of the family. In this vein, we are compelled to expand family research to include family forms that are relevant to this decade. The more traditional family may decline in numbers, but will persist for at least another two generations. At the same time, new family forms, whether identified as wider families, diversified families, postmodern families or any soon-to-be identified new family form, will continue or emerge. The challenge is to adequately research this variation in terms of our culture, our expectations, and personal and interpersonal well-being.

Throughout the past two decades researchers have made the point that the conventional (or traditional) definition of family in the western world is inadequate. The point has been made! We need not hesitate to expand family or marriage definitions by names such as same-sexed parents (SSP) or para families where sexuality is not practiced between the partners (sister and brother, or two friends co-residing), or a grandparent raising a grandchild.

To some, emotional bonds are critical, while to others blood ties are important, and to still others financial support or residence is significant. Eichler's (1990) multi-dimensions of family are relevant. As in other conceptual terms, the family researcher will define the use of the term for the purposes of the research. A universal definition of family at this time will meet with opposition by individuals, the public, law and policy makers, and law enforcers. We can live (and do research) with this ambiguity. The application of this principle will yield scientific and heuristic benefits, leading us to set boundaries for a family definition that is more inclusive than what has been held. It may also produce a more appropriate fit for a family definition at some future point in time.

REFERENCES

Ahrons, C. R. (1979). The binuclear family: Two households, one family. *Alternative Lifestyles, 2*, 499-515.

Aversa, A., Jr. (1991). Neptune yacht club: A family wider than kin. *Marriage & Family Review, 17*(1/2), 45-61.

Baudrillard, J. (1983). *In the shadow of the silent majorities . . . or the end of the social.* New York: Somiotext(e).

Bernardes, J. (1986). Multidimensional development pathways: A proposal to facilitate the conceptualization of A family diversity." *Sociological Review, 34*, 590-610.

Cheal, D. (1991). *Family and the state of theory.* Toronto: U. of Toronto Press.
Cheal, D. (1993). Unity and difference in postmodern families. *Journal of Family Issues, 14*(1), 5-19.
Collier, J. M., Rosaldo, M., & Yanagisko, S. (1982). Is there a family?. In B. Thorne & M. Yalom (Eds.), *Rethinking the family.* New York: Longman.
Coontz, S. (1992, Nov. 15). When a family falls apart: For adult children the trauma can be long-lasting. Baltimore Sun, p. 1F, 2F.
Coser, R. L. (1964). (Ed.). The family: Its structures and functions. New York: St. Martin's Press.
Cowan, C. P., & Cowan, P. A. (1987). Men's involvement in parenthood. In P. W. Berman & F. A. Pederson (Eds.), *Men's transitions to parenthood: Longitudinal studies of early family parenthood* (pp. 145-174). Hillsdale: Lawrence Erlbaum.
Eichler, M. (1990). *Families in Canada To-day.* Toronto: Gage.
Gittins, D. (1986). A feminist look at family development theory. In D. Klein & J. Aldous (Eds.), *Social stress and family development,* (pp. 79-101). New York: Guildford.
Hofferth, S. (1985). Children's life course: Family structure and living arrangements in cohort perspective. In G. Elder (Ed.), Life course dynamics: Trajectories and transitions, 1968-1980 (pp. 75-112). Ithaca, Cornell U. Press.
Larson, L., Goltz, J. W., & Hobart, C. W. (1994). *Families in Canada.* Scarborough, Ont: Prentice Hall.
Levy-Shiff, R., & Israelashvila, R. (1988). Antecedents of fathering: Some further exploration. *Development Psychology, 24,* 434-440.
Marciano, T., & Sussman. M. B. (1991), Wider families: An overview. *Marriage & Family Review, 12*(1/2) 1-8.
MacDonald, L. P., Hornich, J. P., Robertson, G. B., & Wallace, J. E. (1991). *Elder abuse and neglect in Canada.* Toronto: Butterworths.
Murdock, G. P. (1949). Social structure. New York: Macmillan.
Orthner, D. (1995). Families in transition: Changing values and norms. In R. Day, K. Gilbert, B. H. Settles, & W. Burr (Eds.), *Research and Theory in Family Science* (pp. 3-19). New York: Brooks-Cole.
Peters, J. F. (1995). Canadian families in the year 2000. *International Journal of Sociology of the Family, 25,* 63-79.
Pillemer, K. & Finkelhor, D. (1988). The prevalence of elder abuse: A random sample survey. *The Gerontologist, 28,* 51-57.
Rapoport, R. (1989). Ideologics about family forms: Toward diversity. In K. Boh, M. Bak, C. Clason, M. Rankratova, J. Quortup, G. Sgritta, & K. Waerness (Eds.), *Changing patterns of European family life* (pp. 53-69). New York: Routledge.
Scanzoni, J. (1995). Contemporary families and Relationships. New York: McGraw-Hill.
Scanzoni, J., & Marsiglio, W. (1995). Wider families as primary relationships. *Marriage & Family Review, 17*(1/2), 117-133.
Smith, D. (1993). SNAF as an ideological code. *Journal of Family Issues, 14,* 50-65.
Stacey, J. (1990). *Brave new families.* New York: Basic Books.
Stephens, W. N. (1963). The family in cross-cultural perspective. New York: Holt Rinehart & Winston.

Political Systems and Responsibility for Family Issues: The Case of Change in Lithuania

Irena Juozeliuniene

INTRODUCTION

The differences between the responsibility of the totalitarian and the post-Soviet societies in addressing family issues have been dramatically seen in the recent political changes in Lithuania. The usual scholarly observations about close family-society relations seem to be rather banal compared to the social construction of reality, which was central to the examination of the relationship within family units. When conceptualizing the family as a micro-model of a definite type of collectivity (community, state, nation) current Lithuanian family studies raise more questions than they provide answers.

THE FAMILY IN A TOTALITARIAN SOCIETY

In order to understand change a review of how family was viewed in totalitarian society is necessary. Two aspects are especially important: (1) the image of the family as a type of "Soviet collectivity," and (2) a portrait of the Soviet Lithuanian family from the viewpoint of responsibility.

Family as a "Soviet Collectivity"

A brief description of the concepts of "typical" and "ideal type" of the family in the social context is given. Bernardes (1985) uses Mannheim's "total conception of ideology," and states that

Irena Juozeliuniene is affiliated with the Lithuanian Institute of Philosophy and Sociology, Donelaicio 10-2, Vilnius 2009, Lithuania.

[Haworth co-indexing entry note]: "Political Systems and Responsibility for Family Issues: The Case of Change in Lithuania." Juozeliuniene, Irena. Co-published simultaneously in *Marriage & Family Review* (The Haworth Press, Inc.) Vol. 28, No. 3/4, 1999, pp. 67-77; and: *Concepts and Definitions of Family for the 21st Century* (ed: Barbara H. Settles et al.) The Haworth Press, Inc., 1999, pp. 67-77. Single or multiple copies of this article are available for a fee from The Haworth Document Delivery Service [1-800-342-9678, 9:00 a.m. - 5:00 p.m. (EST). E-mail address: getinfo@haworthpressinc.com].

the very existence of 'The Family' seems to be part of the 'total structure of the mind' of contemporary society in much the same way as
notions of ownership and wage labor seems to be. In a dominant ideology, which legitimates current economic and social structure, there is
incorporated a total conception of "family ideology."

In the history of family sociology, there is a significant interest on conceptualizing the family and family-state relations in terms of cultural and
societal perspectives. The totalitarian way of social organization of society
contains many characteristic features but the one of interest for this analysis
is the theme of responsibility in the social context. This theme concerns the
issues of centralization in various spheres of human life that form the understanding of collective identity. The totalitarian social order incorporated the
idea that central managing and direct control would achieve a vision of reality
that was ideologically based. The issue of responsibility was central to the
socialist-communist construction of reality as based on direct moral fundamentalism.

Moral fundamentalism had its roots in the concept of a "Soviet Union."
The "Soviet people" were seen as a unique type of collectivity, different
from those in non-totalitarian countries. Self-designation of individual members of collectivity is an important element in the existence of a stable collectivity. Grosby (1993:5) argues that " . . . this self-designation contributes to
the existence and the continuation of a collectivity by being an object of
attention of the individual members of collectivity. As such, this object unites
the members of the collectivity to one another and to the collectivity itself."
To the extent that a self-designation of the "Soviet people" took place and
the recognition of the shared object existed, then we may speak of the existence of a collective self-consciousness. This process is thought of to be the
basis for development of moral fundamentalism within totalitarian ideology.

Further, so-called "centers" that unite a number of individuals into members of a collectivity must have meaningful referents. Usually, these characteristics convey criteria that determine membership and, as such, contain an
understanding of the jurisdiction of the center. Such a concept of a "Soviet
family" as an elementary unit of the "Soviet society" and the "Soviet
people" maintains the characteristic features of the "center." The "Soviet"
family contained within it various dogmatic values in gender roles, interrelations between spouses, child-parents and family-state relations. It can be
argued that other previous sociological theories about family life had been
based upon the notion of a "typical" pattern or "ideal type" of family.
Bernardes (1981) estimated that at least two hundred "subtle variation" and
diversities of a "typical" family have been observed. The family was assumed to be a necessary condition for the survival and stability of any society, as elementary unit of society, as a vital environment for socialization, and

finally, as the only one "normal" form of family life, all other forms being deviant, pathological and unworkable (Skolnick & Skolnick, 1974). The "Soviet family" model includes some general assumptions based on the family models, as presented by western scholars, for example the "nuclear family model" (Skolnick & Skolnick, 1974).

However, some basic distinctions have to be drawn. The dogmatic values of the "Soviet family" model and the bonds of responsibility within it had nothing in common with the "romantic images of the family" as a highly romanticized version of the past (Settles, 1987, 1992), nor with an image of the "normal" or "typical" family (Skolnick & Skolnick, 1974), presented by scholars in the process of theoretical research. The "Soviet family" sought to create a definite image of exemplary family, containing meaningful referents and criteria of perfect responsibility and accountability. In this ideologically-based image the priority of state affairs took precedence over private needs. Even in the years of "perestroika" in the former Soviet Union, Hartman (1994) noted the amazing lack of privacy in the Soviet family. She stressed that "while Americans emphasize the importance of individuality, personal rights, and privacy, Soviets have been steeped in the belief that society is primary, and they do not even have an exact word for 'privacy'" (p. 7). This ideal model of the family was supported by a variety of means for implementing control which frequently resembled forced efforts to manage a reality according to a priori and dogmatic values.

Conceptualizing Soviet Lithuanian Family and Responsibility

The notion of the "Soviet Lithuanian" family was rarely regarded as being a separate issue because of a clear vision of a "Soviet family" as an ideological "center." Recognition of the Lithuanian family tended to focus on beliefs supporting a particular form of a small unit of society, which was responsible for the reproduction and socialization of members of society (Gurova, 1984; Chartchev, 1979). Attention was given to the varied and multi-layered system of ideas and practices that held that the family was to be a self-sufficient and emotionally balanced environment, which was responsible for bringing up children in the socialist way of life (Markova, 1978). The particularities of the Soviet collectivity caused the same theoretical frameworks and methodology to be applied for family studies, employment collectives, schools and research teams.

This approach yielded a full circle of complex responsibility with accountability: everyone for everyone, parents for children, children for parents, sisters for brothers and vice versa. This accountability of parents to the official institutions (kindergartens, schools, etc.) for the purposeful socialization of a "new type" of a person was taken to extremes according to Vladas Gaidys (1991):

- Everyone in the family unit was made responsible for the political views and activities of the others; the political activities of every adult member of the family were registered in special questionnaires.
- Schools and pre-school establishments as representatives of the Soviet family ideology were made responsible for the upbringing of children. They had a right to influence all activities within the family, especially the control and elimination of religious traditions in the family and the implementation of atheistic ideas and the official vision of the communist society.
- Family life was declared open to the society and controlled by it; the family had to correspond the ideal type of the "Soviet family." The control was exercised in both moral and legal means. One of the spouses had a right to bear a complaint at the workplace, against the other spouse, for example, in the case of hard drinking, adultery, etc. Social institutions were obliged to choose the means of punishment for the sake of the harmony of the family (Gaidys, 1991).

The attempts of the state to penetrate into the family life changed the traditional responsibility within the family. In the socialist society, a comprehensive process of delegation of various functions of a family to the state was undertaken. Issues of sex relations, adultery, divorce, prostitution, suicide were beyond debate. The attitude prevailed that because a high level of morality was a significant characteristic feature of socialist society, it was incompatible with acknowledging the existence of prostitution, divorce, or adultery. Abortions were tolerated on the quiet, since the low birth rate in Lithuania was controlled mainly by abortions as contraceptive means were not easily available. Likewise statistics on suicide were not accessible. Suicide was rejected on the basis of the official statement that "there are no reasons for suicide in socialist society."

Paternalism in Family-State Relations

Paternalism functioned at the center of the Soviet collectivity revealed by state assistance for the family and its relationship to a centrally planned economy. Family policy in Lithuania was not oriented towards establishing conditions to enable families to function independently, or to combine work with family life. The whole employment and pay system and expansion of credits for families maintained a paternalistic state-family relationship. Constant broadening of grants did not encourage the family toward independence and self-responsibility for family's welfare.

In 1988, a national sociological survey (N = 2,800) of working urban and rural populations was undertaken by the Public Opinion Research Center. The 81-item questionnaire was distributed via personnel departments and by mail. The study found that respondents under 30 showed a preference for financial support from the state and better housing instead of improving employment opportunities.

Another aspect of paternalism is avoiding responsibility and delegating it to the state. Morkuniene (1991) suggests several negative consequences on family life by these tendencies:

1. Families tended to avoid responsibility for the upbringing of children, taking care of parents, improving the family welfare.
2. Individuals tended to be indifferent and obedient persons, who were easy to manage in families. This is particularly revealed in the style of behavior of women, who pretend to be mediocre and obedient rather than intelligent; beauty was considered to be important for the sake of the "family welfare."

Individuals were not concerned about the future, or about the issues of child abuse or violence in the family (Morkuniene, 1991).

Because of the notion of their privilege and the stereotyping of behavior of males, there was a pseudo-responsibility by official ideology that influenced the value system. Obedient husbands, accustomed to being ignored and having freedom of choice rather than following the instructions of the state, used to demand the traditional family life. Therefore, the impact on their lifestyle resulted in the drastic modification of responsibility within the whole family.

Women's Situation

Sociological studies of the women's employment and gender roles have been reviewed by Kanopiene (1983). Under the Soviet regime, women were accorded an equal role in the work place. They were expected to engage in paid public work. Ideologically, their high economic activity was promoted as one of the main arguments for sexual equality and the most important precondition of women's liberation from domestic slavery. More practically speaking, economic growth in the Soviet Union (and Lithuania as well) was based on quantitative expansion of the labor force and thus, depended heavily on the contribution of women in the paid labor force. It is necessary to point out that women's employment was stimulated by the socio-economic policies of the state; legislation assuring women's equal rights and equal opportunities with men in education and training for paid work. There was also a broad ideological propaganda aimed at creating a negative image of non-working persons as parasites who were a burden on the community. Women's participation in the labor force was not a matter of option, but of obligation. There was no possibility to choose a different life-style.

These trends in the state-women relations and the subordination of women's domestic responsibilities to the priority of state contradicted the old patriarchal stereotypes in the Lithuanian society. Women were in a psychological crossroad, either giving a priority to the role of motherhood, or to contribution in the development of the welfare of the Soviet collectivity. A functioning powerful "center" left no possibilities to choose one's lifestyle. Women have in the last twenty years comprised nearly half of the total labor force. According to the 1989 Population Census data, 81.0% of females and 86.1% of males of working age were gainfully employed, thus women's economic activity did not differ much from men's.

"Soviet collectivity" had a great impact both on family ideology and practice. The totalitarian way of social organization of society usually left few possible options for other lifestyles. Pseudo-responsibility promoted in this family ideology made a certain family lifestyle an obligation. The belief that the priority of society matters prevents raising the important issues of privacy and self-identity within the family unit. The totalitarian state managed to control the family with the ideologically-based images.

FAMILY IN CONTEMPORARY SOCIETY

Distinctions have to be made between post-Soviet, multiethnic Lithuanian society in transition and the modern western states in the discussion of the notions of civic and democratic nations. Different theoretical backgrounds as well as social practice in the governance of community, equality of opportunities, individual rights, etc., have created different concepts of collective, ethnic and personal identities. One would meet many obstacles trying to define contemporary Lithuanian society in the terms of post-modernity. However, optimists now argue about the potential elimination of drastic contrasts in societal development between the East and the West.

Two main concerns have characterized the transition from totalitarian state to a western type of state. First, the trends of decentralization in all spheres of life have affected moral order of society. The main social-structural causes responsible for this transformation in moral order can be found in the consequences of the functional specialization of the major institutional subsystems of modern society. This process of decentralization breaks the dominance of several sacred dogmas: the "one-meaning" criteria of membership and the dimension of incontestable jurisdiction of the "center." When these concepts change, it may lead to the illusion that morality disappears from modern society. Perhaps the point is really that morality simply changes its location. It is found primarily in individual moral disposition and ethics of behavior as well as in moral communication rather than in ideologically based moral institutions. Western societies have emphasized individual values, family values, community values. In this model all units of the society are said to have "values."

Second, decentralization of the moral order of society is followed by increasing tendency toward a new direction of moral influence. These transitions require a different understanding of collectivity and suggest a new interpretation of coexistence in the community. The perspective of increasing interest to one's personality and self-identity becomes a focus of attention. The family is especially important in times of cultural reorganization. Because it is a very adaptable and functional social system, serving as an important buffer between the individual and the changing environment, the family reacts and changes according to the changes in the outside world.

The Lithuanian family is undergoing major, fundamental changes, which many commentators have seen as "destruction" of the family. It is suggested that those changes should be seen as evolutionary development of society having much in common with the trends that occurred in western countries that happened a couple decades earlier.

Several sociological surveys (Arutunayan, 1986; Maddock, Hogan, Anatolyi & Matskovsky, 1994; Matskovsky, 1989) discuss a shift of post-Soviet families toward western democratic values. Changes in demographic indexes, fertility rates, illegitimate birth rates, and increasing cohabitation support that trend. The number of marriages increased steadily and had a peak of 36.3 thousand per year in 1990. However, a decline was observed from a high of 9.7 marriages per 1000 persons to 6.4 marriages per 1000 in 1993 (the lowest marriage rate observed).

Family size also decreased in Lithuania from an average number of 3 children per family in 1960 to 1.67 children per family in 1994. Until 1990, dissolution of marriages was mainly due to divorces, while today dissolution though death of one of the spouses, especially due to accidents, poisonings, injuries, and suicides, is more frequent. These causes of dissolution parallel the increasing rates of criminality, alcohol abuse and poverty in the society. The changes in illegitimate birth rate during the 50 years before 1990 were not significant. Illegitimate births made up from 6% to 7% of total births. Since 1993, illegitimate birth rate now accounts for 9% of births in Lithuania. At the same time it must be noted that those changes in Lithuania are not as pronounced as in the neighboring post-Soviet countries of Latvia with an illegitimacy rate of 23% and Estonia with a rate of 39%.

Historically the state attempted to be the ultimate authority on right and wrong on the moral development of family members in the Soviet system. Recently, as the decentralization process takes place in state and family ideology, families have once again the dominant responsibility for teaching values. The governing centers of responsibility turn toward periphery and away from family units, and personality itself.

Olson and Matskovsky (1994) emphasized democratization of ethics in post-Soviet families. Their work highlights conflicts within culture, particularly between individualism and allegiance to religious institutions. These manifestations of religious diversity, according to the authors, put pressure on families in relation to personal decision making and choices in the religious upbringing of children.

An extraordinary urgent problem is whether freedom of faith in Lithuania and the influence of family involvement in the religious upbringing of their children will result in high quality of childrearing nationally. Currently there is a general tendency to emphasize individualism in post-Soviet states. The resulting democratization of ethics is occurring in the contemporary Lithuanian society, as well. The period of emotional elation, national solidarity, and the priority setting of state affairs after the restoration of independence in 1990 was followed by the dominance of individualism and the priority of private interests versus state-oriented values.

Attitudes Toward Family Life

Families received a high status in the value systems of post-Soviet countries. In the period of social change, sociological surveys, carried out immediately before and after "perestroika" supported the significance of the family and disclosed the preference of the family-oriented values over social and professional values.

A representative study of values among all nationalities in the Soviet Union (including Lithuanians) in 1986 found that "family" was treated as the most important value, followed by "work" and "respect from others" (Arutunayan, 1986). The data from the 1989 survey on *The Family as a Mirror of Public Opinion* (Matskovsky, 1989) confirmed that family was one of the most important values in the period of rapid social change. Family life was seen as the most appropriate lifestyle. Most of the respondents indicated that "every individual should sooner or later get married and have a family."

In late 1994, a representative sample drawn from 370 territorial units in Lithuania was obtained for a sociological study of family that was conducted by the Lithuanian Institute of Philosophy, Sociology and Law. This questionnaire included 297 questions (both closed and open-ended) and was designed to gain an understanding of values among all nationalities in Lithuania. More than a thousand questionnaires, suitable for analysis, were received.

The survey disclosed a complex index of the personal identity of members of the Lithuanian population. Family issues were on the top of hierarchical order of indexes, followed by the dimension of freedom of choice and morality of interpersonal relations. Family issues hold the dominant position in the structure of personal identity of both females and males (Kanopiene & Juozeliuniene, 1995).

Almost every sociological survey on family matters focused attention on either economic, social or psychological and moral aspects of responsibility.

The survey by Matskovsky (1989) and colleagues on Soviet families indicated that of the vast majority (90%+) of respondents feel responsibility for bringing up children and securing their future. Responsibility for children was followed by desire to create a "good" family (86%). The concept of "good" has a moral aspect in itself; it is manifested in a huge responsibility role. The desire to achieve economic well-being and comfort ranked only seventh in that survey, behind issues such as good health, good friends, interesting work.

A survey designed primarily to examine family issues was conducted by the Lithuanian Institute of Philosophy, Sociology and Law in collaboration with the Department of Statistics in 1992-1993. Fifteen hundred questionnaires were received back including 344 by young respondents aged 18-30. Responsibility in family life was analyzed by including questions on divorce, adultery and abortions (Juozeliuniene, 1993). In general, divorce and adultery were treated negatively, but divorce was tolerated to a larger extent. At a more subtle and complex level the respondents disclosed their values on holding family units together. Respect of the rights of a partner as well as dignity were two main responsibility values. Next came the influence of interrelations between spouses on upbringing children in the family, particularly on self-esteem and self-respect of a child. Having a comfortable environment in family life by avoiding hard drinking, adultery, etc., was also important.

Family life is defined as a phenomenon with the main characteristics of providing emotional comfort of all family members as well as self-security, self-importance and self-pride. For that reason Lithuania still remains a country with rather stable, traditional, married nuclear families. Other forms of living together, such as cohabitation, "living apart together," etc., are not so widespread as in other European countries. However, when family life loses its function of moral and emotional support and when self-security cannot be ensured by the means of family life, it is not worth living together.

The examination of the attitudes toward adultery leads to the interesting conclusion that adultery is tolerated and even approved when daily routine and lack of fascinating perspectives in family life are found. The second most common reason for justifying adultery is falling in love with another person. Sexual incompatibility (difficulties in intimate life) was the third most common justification for adultery. Thus, the abilities of a couple not to give way to daily routine evidently lie in the center of their ability to prevent adultery.

The primary reason given for justifying abortion was a consideration of the fate of unwanted and unloved children. The second most important reason given was anxiety about woman's health; the third a lack of a successful means of birth control. Keep in mind that the children's affairs were treated by respondents as sufficient reason to divorce as well as to commit abortions. Child-related problems are close to the center of family values.

The mere fact that we now can do research and scholarly study on the "prohibited" aspects of the family life, demonstrates the end of the era of "Soviet collectivity." With the end of that concept, centralization of moral order of society as well as the direction of moral influence has shifted toward the development of identity of the family and individual identities of the family members. Obviously, families in Lithuania came to have the dominant responsibility for teaching values and responsibility.

While theoretical conclusions resulting from the recent surveys on family issues hardly could be treated as sufficient and exhaustive background, they provide some clues for the development of post-Soviet family ideology in Lithuania. Many projects on family issues, supported by the official institutions of the state, primarily have in their aim to draw mainly socio-economic and demographic portrait of Lithuanian family in transition and value studies have been beyond the field of interest. However, it must be noted that the value-oriented studies of family issues are becoming part of the agenda. The need to create a theoretical background for family studies, appropriate to the period of transition, is still of a great urgency.

REFERENCES

Arutunayan, Y. V. (Ed.) (1986). *Similarities and differences among ethnic cultures: Sociological images of Soviet Nations.* Moscow.

Bernardes, J. (1981). *Diversity within and alternatives to "The Family": The development of an alternative theoretical approach.* Unpublished doctoral dissertation. University of Hull.

Bernardes, J. (1985). Family ideology: Identification and exploration. *The Sociological Review, 33*(2), 275-297.

Chartchev, A. G. (1979). *Marriage and family in the Soviet Union.* Moscow (in Russian).

Juozeliuniene, I. (1993). *Young people in Lithuania: Social condition and search for a new values.* Paper presented at the Eighth International Congress on Young People. Trento.

Hartman, S. (1994). Introduction. In J. W. Maddock, M. J. Hogan, A. I. Antonov & M. S. Matskovsky (Eds.), *Families before and after perestroika-Russian and U.S. Perspectives* (pp. 1-8). The Guilford Press.

Gaidys, V. (1991). *The sun-town and Lithuanian family: Family and nation.* Vilnius, Lithuania (in Lithuanian).

Grosby, S. (1993). *The significance of nationality.* Paper presented at the Eighth International Congress on Young People, Trento.

Gurova, R. (1984). *Sociological problems of upbringing.* Kaunas, Lithuania (in Lithuanian).

Kanopiene, V. (1983). *Women's labor in Lithuanian SSR.* Vilnius, Lithuania (in Russian).

Kanopiene, V., & Juozeliuniene, I. (1995). *Women in Lithuania: Employment, values, identity.* Paper presented at the fiftieth World Congress of Central and East European studies, Warsaw, Poland.

Maddock, J. W., Hogan, M. J., Antonov, A. I., & Matskovsky, M. S. (Eds.) (1994). *Families before and after perestroika-Russian and U.S. perspectives.* NY: The Guilford Press.

Markova, T. (Ed.) (1987). *Coaching children for school at home.* Kaunas, Lithuania (in Lithuanian).

Matskovsky, M. S. (Ed.) (1989). *The family as a mirror of public opinion.* Report on the survey conducted in collaboration with the All-Union Center for Public Opinion. Vilnius, Lithuania.

Morkuniene, J. (1991). *State and family–the criteria of recognition: Family and nation.* Vilnius, Lithuania (in Lithuanian).

Olson, D. V., & Matskovsky, M. S. (1994). Soviet and American families: A comparative overview. In J. W. Maddock, M. J. Hogan, A. I. Antonov & M. S. Matskovsky (Eds.), *Families before and after perestroika-Russian and U.S. Perspectives* (pp. 9-35). The Guilford Press.

Settles, B. H. (1987). A perspective on tomorrow's families. In M. B. Sussman, & S. K. Steinmetz (Eds.), *Handbook of Marriage and the Family* (pp. 157-180). NY: Plenum.

Settles, B. H. (1992). *Issues for Family Sociologists.* Paper presented at the 29th CFR Seminar, Vilnius, Lithuania.

Skolnick, A. S., & Skolnick J. H. (1974). *Domestic relations and social change: Intimacy, family and society.* Boston: Little Brown.

Family as a Set of Dyads

Jan Trost

INTRODUCTION

From my perspective, one could say that there are four more or less divergent or different kinds of definitions that can be applied to the concept of family. Any phenomenon within social reality could be dealt with in a similar way and families are certainly not unique in this respect.

Defining Family

The four kinds of definitions that can be used to define family:

1. *Theoretical or nominal definitions.* These are aimed at being used in our theoretical or model building efforts and are also involved in operational definitions.

Jan Trost is affiliated with the Department of Sociology, University of Uppsala, Box 513, Uppsala, Sweden.

[Haworth co-indexing entry note]: "Family as a Set of Dyads." Trost, Jan. Co-published simultaneously in *Marriage & Family Review* (The Haworth Press, Inc.) Vol. 28, No. 3/4, 1999, pp. 79-91; and: *Concepts and Definitions of Family for the 21st Century* (ed: Barbara H. Settles et al.) The Haworth Press, Inc., 1999, pp. 79-91. Single or multiple copies of this article are available for a fee from The Haworth Document Delivery Service [1-800-342-9678, 9:00 a.m. - 5:00 p.m. (EST). E-mail address: getinfo@haworthpressinc.com].

2. *Operational definitions.* This label is confusing sometimes because these definitions are simply forms of measurement such as the questions composing a questionnaire. When operational definitions are used, one should also have a theoretical definition of the particular phenomenon as a guide. The operational definition ideally should be concerned with exactly the same construct as the theoretical one; otherwise the validity will be low and less congruence will exist between what is intended to be measured and what is actually assessed.

3. *Phenomenological definitions.* Under these definitions, we step outside of our ivory towers and confront ourselves with the human social beings in which we are interested. We could, for example, simply ask our research participants what they perceive as their family or to report what they see as the meaning of family more generally. Levin (1990), for example, has dealt with one way of collecting and analyzing phenomenological definitions.

4. *Empirical definitions.* Empirical definitions are based on our interest in determining what people do in connection with the term family. More specifically, the concept is more or less defined by the behavior of people, not how they conceptualize, but what they demand and expect of members' activities. These demands and expectations control inclusion and exclusion of family members. Gubrium and Holstein's work (1990) is an example of defining family in an empirical manner.

Phenomenological and empirical definitions have a lot in common. If we want to understand the mechanisms behind the inclusion and exclusion of persons in the individual's concept of their own family, the person's expectations and the other's behavior will assist in our understanding.

Nominal or theoretical definitions have been in the forefront of thinking about families for a considerable amount of time along with various ways of operationalizing them. Settles (1987), for example, indicates that not only are there numerous varieties of theoretical definitions, the chance for complete agreement about "what is family" is very small or non-existent. I agree a lot but not totally, and also feel comfortable in believing that we do not have to agree. In fact, I would even go so far as to claim that we should not agree. Furthermore, the traditional way of defining family should be challenged. In the long run, however, we might come to an agreement about what sort of "language" to use when distinguishing one variety of family from another.

Murdock (1949) defined a nuclear family as a man and a woman, living in an emotional, economic, and sexual relationship, and their children. With his approach, he could divide all sorts of families from various cultures into sets of nuclear families. A polyandrous family was defined as consisting of (1) one nuclear family constituted by the woman and one of her husbands plus their common children, and (2) one nuclear family constituted by the woman and another of her husbands and their common children, etc. In a similar way, an extended family would consist of a number of nuclear families from different generations who are living together in the same household.

The concept of family can be deconstructed in a similar manner and, in the spirit of Georg Simmel, I will take the dyad as the basic unit of analysis (Trost 1988, 1990). In a manner similar to the way that nuclear families can be combined into more complex units, for example, parent-child units and spousal units can be combined in various ways. Consequently, the smallest single-parent family would be defined as a family consisting of one dyad only: the parent-child dyad, or the child-parent dyad, if you wish. The smallest "nuclear" family would consist of three dyads: one spousal dyad, one mother-child dyad, and one father-child dyad. The smallest three-generation family, if conceptualized from the perspective of a child, would consist of (1) a grandparent-parent dyad, (2) a child-parent dyad, and (3) a grandchild-grand-parent dyad.

Similarly, a married couple with two children can be viewed as one spousal unit (husband and wife) and four parent-child units (mother with each child and father with each child). In everyday language these family components constitute a two-parent, two-child family and, when all live together, a household is constituted.

One household is divided into two households when a married couple divorces or a married or cohabiting couple separates. In this case, if only one child lives exclusively with one of the parents who is the physical custodian, traditional terminology would define this as a one-parent family. This would mean, of course, that the non-custodial parent would clearly not be a member of the single-parent family, but instead, constitute a single-person household. In contrast, from my own viewpoint, the custodial parent and the child might constitute a parent-child unit, and a household; the non-custodial parent and the child also constitute a parent-child unit, but not a household. Moreover, we might be defining two families here if, in the example above, both parents have joint custody.

Using traditional language, I might say that the three persons make two one-parent families. At any given moment, such circumstances mean that one single-parent family exists, defined by where the child lives at the moment, and one single-person household exists. Two households would exist, which alternate periodically, depending upon the location of the child. With the approach offered here, one would simply conclude that there are two parent-child units. Such is the case, even if the child remains with one parent, but both adults continue to be parents, even if their spousal relationship has disappeared. The child still has two parents and, therefore, two families may exist. However, the parents and child might differ in how they construct their circumstances after a separation or divorce has occurred.

Let us look at another case. Two women cohabit and they each have one child from previous relationships who reside with them. Therefore, a four-person household is constituted which might be classified by society as two single-parent families sharing a household, but not commonly viewed as a two-parent family. If a man and a woman cohabit or are married and they have one resident child each from previous relationships, several interpretations are possible. They live in a four-person household, which might be classified either as (1) a spousal unit and two single-parent families who share a household or (2) a two-parent family. From the dyadic perspective presented here, in both cases, only two parent-child units exist in each household unless the noncustodial parent assumes, socially and otherwise, a parental role relationship in reference to the child.

Taking over a parental role relationship should not be taken for granted, as is often the case within census and other demographic studies of households My own view, however, is that such relationships should be individually examined and not taken for granted. From a dyadic perspective, any type of hyphenated-family or other family form could be easily defined, regardless of whether the aim is scientific or political. Consequently, I agree with Liss (1987:796) who says: "Rather than settling for a particular definition, it seems more appropriate to define families according to the particular issues involved."

My approach with dyadic units was first developed at a small informal seminar in Belgium (Trost 1988). Since then it has been applied to empirical data collected both quantitatively and qualitatively. Several examples of these applications of the theoretical ideas with the dyads have been used to illustrate its utility. While these initial applications are rather straightforward and would need to be culturally adapted for various societies with different legal and traditional usage of family, they are useful in helping us to see how readily one can find different perceptions in fairly homogenous cultures.

WHAT DOES SOCIAL REALITY MEAN BY FAMILY?

In order to see how the phenomenon of the family is conceptualized I will briefly present two sets of data; one quantitative, the other qualitative.

Quantitative Data

During the spring of 1989 a questionnaire was sent by mail to a statistically representative sample of 1,500 persons aged 20-59 years in the Uppsala province of Sweden. After some reminders, we received 935 questionnaires, producing a response rate of 62% of those sampled.

One of the questions requested the respondent to list all those individuals whom he or she counted as members of their own family. The respondents were informed that I was not interested in participants' names, but in the specific relationships each member occupied in reference to the respondent. Another question contained a number of examples of family constellations, with each respondent being asked to indicate whether they considered each constellation to be a family.

This latter question is a further development of what Gilby and Pedersen (1982) have used. Because we, as scholars, do not know or agree about what is meant by the term family, I first wanted to ascertain how the members of the general population empirically define their own families. Next, I was interested in the more general concept of family when respondents do not connect this construct to their own social and familial situation. Furthermore, I suggest that their empirical definitions can be interpreted as showing the respondents' internal theories or principles that underlie their responses.

The respondents were asked: "When you think upon *your* family, who are you thinking about: Write each one on each line?" The answers have been conservatively coded so that if, for example, "brothers" was written on a single line instead of using one line per brother (so that it was not possible to know how many brothers the respondent meant to include), this was coded as two. This means that the number of family members, in most cases, is exactly what the respondent has indicated; when this is not clear, our estimates are the lowest possible number. The responses, including the respondent varied from 0 to 40 members. The median was 5.0 and the mode was 4.0 family members, with 20 percent of the participants' responses being consistent with the mode.

Most of the respondents reported that their families consisted of a spouse/cohabitant and/or a child or children. Fewer included a parent or parents, but more than a third included sibling(s). An even smaller number included grandchildren, children's spouses/cohabitants, parent(s)-in-law, stepparent(s), step-child(ren), sibling's spouses, sibling's children, ex-spouse/cohabitant, friend(s), and pet(s).

When we inquire about the respondent's family, the variety is enormous, not only in terms of the number of members, but also in reference to the types of relationships. Some include only nuclear family members, while others broaden their definitions of family to include at least some of the kin. Such tendencies to broaden the definition of one's own family involves combining legal/social connections with those based in conjugality along with such biological connections as consanguinity. A few even include other categories such as friends and pets.

The respondents were then provided with examples of units of two or more individuals and asked to respond with either "yes" or "no" to the question: "Which of the enumerated groups are families according to your perspective?" The results, indicating the percentage of respondents who defined a particular unit as a "family," are shown on Table 1.

Some clarification might be required. In Sweden, marriage is legally possible only for opposite gender couples. Göran and Greta, Håkan and Hanna, Ingemar and Inger, Martin and Mona, are opposite-gender couples. The same-

TABLE 1. Percent of respondents defining the case as a family.

Anna and Anders are a middle-aged married couple without any children. Are they a family?	75%
Bodil and Bertil are a married couple in their thirties; they have a six-year-old son, Bengt. Are these three a family?	99%
Cecilia is divorced and has a ten year old daughter, Carin, who lives with Cecilia. Are these two a family?	83%
Carin's father, Curt, lives at the other end of the city. Are Curt and Carin a family?	33%
Are Cecilia and Curt a family?	8%
Doris and David are Daniel's maternal grandparents. They do not live together with Daniel. Are these three a family?	23%
Eva and Edvin are married and they have a daughter, named Elisabeth. These three live together. Eva and Edvin have a son, Erik, who lives in another city. Are these four a family?	84%
Fanny and Fredrik are married and have a teenager son, Frans, who has a friend, Sven. All these four live together. Are these four a family?	41%
Göran and Greta are in their thirties and have lived together for three years, they have no children. Are they a family?	60%
Hanna and Håkan are in their thirties and live together, they have a six-year-old daughter, Hedvig. Are these three a family?	97%
Ingemar and Inger have lived together, they are now separated. They have a ten-year-old son, Isak, who lives with Ingemar. Are these three a family?	13%
Isak's mother, Inger, lives at the other end of the city. Are Inger and Isak a family?	34%
Jan, Johanna, and Jesper are siblings and all are in their thirties. The three live together. Are these three a family?	50%
Karl and Krister are in their thirties and live together. No one of them has a child. Are these two a family?	30%
Lena and Lisa are both in their thirties and live together. Lisa has a six-year-old daughter, Lotta. These three live together. Are these three a family?	38%
Mona and Martin are married and they have a daughter around ten years old, Maria. Mona has a very good friend with whom she can talk about anything. Are these four a family?	8%

gender couples are the males Karl and Krister as well as the females Lena and Lisa. All these names are clearly and without a doubt gender-related for a Swede. The Swedish term "sambo" was used in the Swedish questionnaire to refer to relationships like non-marital cohabitation. It is translated in this article as "live together" which is certainly true for opposite-gender couples, but somewhat less likely to have a similar meaning for the same-gender couples.

Almost everyone includes a married or cohabiting couple with children, roughly the nuclear family model, within the concept of family. Most respondents look upon a divorced couple as being individuals who no longer are in the same family. Almost one out of five excludes a single parent living with a child from their concept of family. Phrased somewhat differently, of course, more than four out of five respondents include a single-parent with a child within their concept of family. Many respondents also include a son who is not currently living with his parents (who do live together) within their concept of family.

About one out of three respondents include persons who are partners in a same-gender couple within their concept of family. I do not know, however, whether the respondents have concluded that the same gender couples are homosexual. I deliberately decided not to refer to homosexuality, because if such a reference were made, I would have likewise been obligated to indicate that the married and cohabiting couples are heterosexual. This would have, of course, seemed foolish but necessary. The Swedish term "sambo" cannot be misunderstood for opposite-gender couples, with non-marital cohabitation being the referent circumstance. A similar connotation is quite likely for the same-gender couples.

When formulated in terms of dyadic units, more popular (in number of respondents) family constellations have the following order of respondent identification: (1) the combination of a spousal or cohabiting unit, two parent-child units, and a common domicile (the B's and the H's with 99% and 97% respectively); (2) a spousal (or cohabitational?) unit and parent-child units where a common domicile is not necessary (the E's with 84% of the "vote"); (3) a parent-child unit and a common domicile (Cecilia and her daughter, 83%); (4) a spousal unit that, by definition, involves an opposite-gender relationship (the A's, 75%); (5) a cohabitational unit involving an opposite-gender relationship (the G's with 60%), and (6) sibling units having a common domicile (the J's, 50%).

When delimiting the meaning of "family" for others rather than for themselves, therefore, it seems evident that domicile is an important dimension for quite a few of the above categories. Also high on the list of important dimensions are spousal and parent-child units.

Qualitative Data

Qualitative data also was collected using a method developed by Levin (1989, 1990; see also her article in this volume) that enables people to define their own family. Specifically, the interviewer asks the respondent to write the names of their own family members on a slip of paper. When this is completed, the interviewer asks each respondent to place the members of the family on a big sheet of paper using small pieces of paper symbolizing the members, where circular pieces symbolize females, and triangular pieces symbolize males. The third step is to ask respondents about the meaning of the depicted spatial arrangements on the sheet; what categories are included or excluded, and what the distance between the symbols means. Thus, the data gathered consists of the picture on the big sheet and the interview.

In one of my previous studies, I used only the first two steps, the list and the picture, omitting the interview. At an international colloquium, I asked the participants at one session to list their own family members, and glue the picture of their family to a sheet of paper. After some opposition they complied. The results were similar to the quantitative study in demonstrating the following categories: (1) nuclear family members, spouse and children, but no one else, (2) household members who were not nuclear family members, (3) parents, (4) parents-in-law, (5) children's spouses or "friends" (probably indicating cohabitants or fiancées), (6) grandchildren (7) siblings (8) a mistress (9) an ex-spouse, (10) friends, and (11) pets.

An elderly person was very sad, for example, because she had no family, but after a while she asked if she would be allowed to define herself and her dog as her family. She did, and found, that after all, even she and her dog were a family. One of the respondents indicated at another time that family consisted of parents, siblings, friends, and music, a result indicating that even immaterial phenomena can be included in one's notion of family.

Another informant, a divorced mother of two children, provided a different perspective. She placed herself and the children in the middle of the sheet, but also placed a sister, the sister's husband, and their two children near her. The geographic distance is substantial but the emotional distance is small and, therefore, the sister is placed close on the sheet. The sister-in-law is included despite the fact that the respondent does not like her, and she feels that it would be unfair or an injustice to exclude her. Moreover, she places her ex-husband, of whom she is not at all fond, relatively close to her. He lives close by, however, and is included as a family member for the children's sake. Thus, the spatial distance reflects a combined representation of geographic distance, emotional distance, and her wish for a close relationship between her children and their father.

An immigrant refugee represented his family by listing the symbols for his mother, his two sisters, and his three brothers, but left himself out. When asked where he had listed himself, he simply stated that he was "here," making clear that he referred to living in Sweden. Specifically, he meant that he has no family of procreation, but does have a family of orientation, with his father being deceased. However, he has not seen members of his family of orientation for many years, and since he has not been allowed or able to see his mother or siblings for such a long period, he does not consider himself to be a member of his own family. If, or when, he returns to his family he will then automatically renew his family membership.

An important conclusion from these qualitative studies is concerned with the question "what dyads would be included in the individual's conceptualization?" Three sorts of dyads seem to be apparent:

1. The individual is one of the members in a given dyad and not only in some of the dyads but possibly in all of them.
2. Some of the other persons in a dyad with the individual can also form other dyads together (i.e., from the individual's definition). For example, the mother and the father might be defined as a dyad but possibly components of three dyads: the individual and the mother, the individual and the father, the mother and the father.
3. A person who is *not* in any of the individual's dyads could be in a dyad with someone who is a member of one of the individual's dyads. An example would be a mother who views herself as (1) being in a dyad with a child, (2) but does not define the father of her child as being in one of her own dyads, and yet (3) defines the child and father as a separate dyad within her family.

IMPLICATIONS

When asked, quite a few respondents would label a household of an adult couple with three children as a family. This seems very simple, but when asked to tell us what their own family looks like, as demonstrated above, the responses of participants are likely to fall into at least five different categories. Qualitative data reveal that some would stress consanguinity, others conjugality, while some would emphasize the principle of a common domicile. A few do not emphasize these limitations and accept a surprisingly wide variety of social groupings to be families.

The qualitative data also reflect that a wide variety of meanings are linked to the term family. Common basic units or dyads are referred to such as spousal units, cohabitational units, parent-child units, master-dog units, sibling units, and ex-spousal units. Some individuals actively *exclude* persons, who according to alternative principles that might be used, should be members, by presumably invoking another principle that allows the person to be excluded. Similarly, some persons are actively *included*, even if one principle might not include them because another principle is given priority in the mind of the respondent. Consider, for example, the ex-husband who was not liked and did not "really belong to my family," but is included because he is the children's father. Or the sister-in-law who also was not liked, but was included because it "would be an injustice" not to include her when another sister-in-law is included. In such cases, a principle of justice seems to have superseded kinship and emotional principles.

Another pattern was that respondents listed pets and included them in the family pictures in such countries as Sweden, France, the USA, Hong Kong, and Japan. This does not mean that no differences exist between these cultures or societies, but that similarity of this kind is important in understanding the meaning of family.

Although in the introduction I indicated that I would not try to define family, in effect, I have implicitly suggested that groups consisting of at least one parent-child unit and/or at least one spousal unit may, indeed, be a family. These two definitions, however, are only examples of definitions of small families.

Let me illustrate how this dyadic approach could be used in developing research or social policy. Assume that our aim, for example, is to look at the housing situation for what in vernacular is referred to as a single-parent family.

Traditionally, we reasonably might restrict the definition of a one-parent family to one or more parent-child unions who live in one household but do not have a spousal unit. By doing so, of course, we would exclude situations where the parent and the child(ren) do not live together, where the parent has (re)married, and where the parent has begun to cohabit.

In some countries, social policies are aimed at supporting and simplifying the contacts between parents and children, even if they are not living together. This can mean that society provides some housing subsidies to a noncustodial parent so that a child can stay with the parent during such time periods as week-ends and vacations. Such circumstances may make it reasonable to talk about non-residential single-parent families. These families would then be defined as at least a one parent-child unit without a common domicile. Depending on the particular aim, instances where the non-residential parent has formed a spousal unit might be taken into consideration as well.

I hope these examples have demonstrated that the approach described here would clarify the meaning of family as well as the data collection, analysis, and application efforts. One person is not a family, but a variety of groups can be a family consisting of a number of subgroups. Many possible definitions exist that can carry valid meanings. The law can define what a family is, and does so with varying precision and with varying content, dependent upon the aim of the law. Practitioners such as family physicians, family therapists, and pediatricians, just to mention a few, can define what a family means for them and also of what the client's family consists. Scholars can define what a family is from a theoretical as well as from an empirical standpoint, while individuals can define for themselves of what their own family consists.

The smallest unit of a family group is a couple, dyad, or pair that can take the specific form of a married couple or parent-child dyad. Such families would include a married couple with a child or a spousal unit and two parent-child units (a number of children and other related persons can be added). Those included are limited by conjugality, that is, legally defined marital relationships, in-law relationships, or in terms of consanguinity (i.e., blood or biological relatedness). I would not, of course, limit the concept family to these ideas, but instead, recognize that many possibilities exist–controlled by our ideologies and our tastes.

FORMATION AND REFORMATION

A family is *formed, according to my definition*, when a couple (i.e., two persons) either marries or, in the case of cohabitation, moves in together. The other means of *forming* a family occurs when a child is born and taken care of by a single parent or a couple.

If spouses have a child, a family is *not* formed. Such a family already exists and the addition of a child or subsequent children means simply that the family is being *reformed* or *reformulated*. Similarly, when a single woman with a child marries or begins to cohabit with a man or woman (whether the father of the child or someone else), the existing family might transition from being a two-member into a three-member family.

Liljeström and Kollind (1990) use the same term, in Swedish, *ombildad familj*, which literally means a "reformed family." They use this term, however, to avoid the term "step" family for those who have married, begun to cohabit, or where at least one of the spouses/partners has a previous child living in the common household. I am also not an advocate of using the term "step" family in today's society and my use of the term "reformed" family differs from that used by Liljeström and Kollind. Specifically, my use of the term indicates a change or a process, while Liljeström and Kollind use the term for a circumstance after the change (i.e., a more static way indicating a state). Duberman (1975), for example, uses the term "reconstituted family" in a somewhat similar manner and, as far as I can see, she uses this term to designate step-family constellations. From my perspective, however, she refers to a state, but does not designate the concept of process. Furthermore, in most or maybe even all cases, a family already exists that just adds one or more persons. As a result, the family is simply being reformed and not being reconstituted.

Remarriages and recohabitations can be formations of new families, but most are simply reformations. Even if a divorced or widowed person has only adult children who do not live at home and the person remarries, their family is not being formed. Much of the meaning of formation and reformation, of course, depends upon whose glasses one is looking through.

CONCLUSION

The system of dyadic units used when defining and conceptualizing a family also provides, as a side effect, another perspective (Trost, 1993, 1996). Not only is it reasonable to be concerned about the use of such terms as formation and reformation, but this perspective also broadens what a family is considered to be. Moreover, we rapidly and almost automatically raise the issue and concern about who is doing the defining–the theoretician, researcher, supervisor, therapist, and the individual, etc.? Consequently, we should not take any perspective for granted when we know that an enormous variety of perspectives exists (Trost, 1995).

Another side effect of the dyadic approach has to do with the phenomenon of defining family. Many agree that we should not define *the* family and recognize that we can only define varieties of families. Some that are referred to as some kind of hyphenated family could be just as well labeled as having some kind of purpose. An important thing here is that we avoid defining any of the hyphenated families as *the hyphenated family form.* To define *the* stepfamily or *the* one-parent family would be normative and thus problematic. But we can report and hence define *a sort of* or *a* kind of stepfamily or one-parent family.

REFERENCES

Duberman, L. (1975). *A reconstituted family: A study of remarried couples and their children.* Chicago: Nelson Hall.

Gilby, R. L., & Pedersen, D. R. (1982). The development of the child's concept of the family. *Canadian Journal of Behaviour Science, 14,* 110-121.

Gubrium, J. F., & Holstein, J A. (1990). *What is family?* Mountain View: Mayfield.

Levin, I. (1989). Hva er en familie? En presentasjon av en metode. *Fokus pd familien, 17,* 25-31.

Levin, I. (1990). How to define family. *Family Reports, 17,* Uppsala University.

Liljeström, R. & Kollind, A. (1990). Kärleksliv och föräldraskap. Stockholm: Carlsson.

Liss, L. (1987). Families and the law. In M. B. Sussman & S. K. Steinmetz (Eds.), *Handbook of Marriage and the Family* (pp. 767-794). New York: Plenum Press.

Murdock, G. P. (1949). *Social structure.* New York: The Free Press.

Settles, B. H. (1987). A perspective on tomorrow's families. In M. B. Sussman & S. K.

Steinmetz (Eds.), *Handbook of Marriage and the Family* (pp. 157-180). New York: Plenum Press.

Trost, J. (1988). Conceptualising the family. *International Sociology, 3*, 301-308.

Trost, J. (1990). Do we mean the same by the concept of family? *Communication Research, 16*, 431-443.

Trost, J. (1993). Family from a dyadic perspective. *Journal of Family Issues, 14*, 92-104.

Trost, J. (1995). Households, families and dissolution. *Scandinavian Population Studies, 10*, 77-88.

Trost, J. (1996). Family structure and relationships: The dyadic approach. *Journal of Comparative Family Studies, 27*, 395-408.

What Phenomenon Is Family?

Irene Levin

INTRODUCTION

The stepfamily challenges traditional definitions of family where family is equated with household and where socialization of children is an important task for the couple. In stepfamilies the complexity of the concept of family is clear in the sense that not all members of the household have the same biological or legal connections to each other. This article describes a method of defining family from the perspective of the individual. While the method was developed in a study of stepfamilies, it can be used for other purposes and with other groups as well.

Defining Family

If one asks a group of persons, "Do you know what *family* is?", the answers will be in the affirmative. We relate to *family* as if there were general agreement on the meaning. In contrast, if one asks the same group, "Who is your family?", the answers often do not demonstrate the same unity. Almost everyone will have different criteria for whom to include, such as those within the household, others, parents, siblings or their partner's kin. For some, death is a way of leaving the family, as divorce has become for some. Friends will be included in their family by a few respondents, while others will not include kin with whom they are not emotionally close.

Some sort of an agreement seems to exist about what family means. At the same time, however, the individual's social construction of family suggests that not only one, but numerous concepts of family exist (Levin, 1994).

Irene Levin is affiliated with Oslo College, Tjernveien 12, 0957 Oslo, Norway.

[Haworth co-indexing entry note]: "What Phenomenon Is Family?" Levin, Irene. Co-published simultaneously in *Marriage & Family Review* (The Haworth Press, Inc.) Vol. 28, No. 3/4, 1999, pp. 93-104; and: *Concepts and Definitions of Family for the 21st Century* (ed: Barbara H. Settles et al.) The Haworth Press, Inc., 1999, pp. 93-104. Single or multiple copies of this article are available for a fee from The Haworth Document Delivery Service [1-800-342-9678, 9:00 a.m. - 5:00 p.m. (EST). E-mail address: getinfo@haworthpressinc.com].

Gubrium and Holstein (1990) characterize this as the difference between *THE family* and *family*–in definite and indefinite form. They write about *THE family* as a more static description of "the thing" family, whereas *family* is a more a processual concept, changing from person to person, according to time and space. For example, Bernardes (see his article in this volume) describes such dilemmas of defining family, while, at the same time, he takes the position that a deeper understanding of family life is needed. He argues, in turn, that in order to do so, scholars should not use a static concept, but must refuse to define *THE family*.

In 1949 Murdock challenged both researchers and nonprofessionals to conduct further analyses about what the term *family* really means. Bell and Vogel (1960) mention the different meanings of family being dependent on individual definitions similar to the manner of Gross (1987) nearly 30 years later. She qualifies her statement, however, by proposing that our knowledge will increase with further research on the concept of family. Settles (1987) is more pessimistic about the future possibilities of developing a single definition when she refers to the many different types of definitions that exist. Specifically, she proposes that "it is not likely that the job of specifying what is meant by *family* will progress rapidly. Consensus would be . . . improbable for scholars" (p. 161).

In everyday language "family" relates to a social group that is biologically, legally and emotionally connected. The concept family can also connote the quality of a relationship much as the word "familiar" means something known to you. Such varied and subtle meanings are seldom referred to in the scientific literature, although a further understanding of everyday use most probably will increase our general understanding of the concept (Rommetveit, 1979; Jorgenson, 1986). For example, Caplow, Bahr, Chadwick, Hill and Williamson (1982) emphasize, in their study of Middletown, that if you say "my family" or "our family," it is unclear whom you include. You can include children not living in the household, but not necessarily. If you say: "my family is coming for Christmas," the persons might not be the same as those whom you include in the statement "the family lives here in Middletown."

The term family stands for many different concepts that are often clarified by such things as the context and one's tone of voice. Family or family relations are often used metaphorically to emphasize if the relationship is positive or negative. For example, the statement "She is like a sister for me" conveys meaning about closeness and responsibilities felt towards another woman. Similarly, the phrase "the group functioned as a family" can convey particularly positive relationships between the group members. Moreover, the tone of the voice is decisive as to how the concept "family" will be understood in the latter sentence. Used with a different tone or in another context, such phrases can convey conflicting meanings.

Many discussions exist which propose that *the family* (i.e., something we all know about and agree upon) will disappear. Moreover, there is much discussion about the future of *the family*, which appears to be based on common agreement about what *the family is* and the assumption that we all see it the same way.

Three Perspectives

Discussion about the definition of family is not new and we are not the first group of scholars who ask this vital and important question. Previously, discussions have dealt mostly with how to define *THE family*. From a societal perspective, scholars such as Parsons (1955), Murdock (1949), Winch (1971), and later Reiss (1987) have provided different types of definitions. Parsons (1955) provides a functional definition that contains two main ideas; the family as stabilizing the adult personality and nurturing children. Murdock (1949), on the other hand, defines family somewhat differently as

> a social group characterized by common residence, economic coopera-
> tion, and reproduction. It includes adults of both sexes, at least two of
> whom maintain a socially approved sexual relationship, and one or
> more children, own or adopted, of the sexually cohabiting adults. (p. 1)

Each "social group" is, for Murdock, like an atom within a molecule. Society consists of numerous atoms or nuclei, and Murdock was the first to introduce the term "nuclear family." Murdock's use of this concept was meant as a societal level descriptor and not, as is often the case today, an application at the small group level of analysis.

For Reiss (1987), the family is "the small kinship group composed of anyone nurturing the newborn," with a child being necessary for a family to exist. From this point of view, a couple without a child does not constitute a family. In a similar manner, Winch (1963) had earlier used a functional definition and described family as the basic social structure that has "replacement" as its primary social function.

Broderick (1987) equates family and household in viewing these concepts from a small group perspective. Family for him involves two or more persons who live in the same household and are related through blood, marriage, or adoption. He excludes other persons living together as family because consanguinity and conjugality are important criteria for membership. For Broderick, one *has to be* kin or married, a definition that excludes cohabitants from being family members. Broderick's definition coincides with how the concept family is often used in everyday language, as being the same as household. It is important to recognize, however, that the term "familia" in Latin also means household. Consequently, the concept "household" includes only kin for Broderick, whereas the Roman term included all those living in the household such as servants, slaves, and various kin.

Family therapists frequently use family in the same manner as Broderick. When client is asked to bring in his or her family for the next session, they expect the rest of the household to show up. The term family has not been seen as a problem by family therapists (Levin, 1989a, 1990), with many not recognizing that extended insight can be provided by a more processual and less normative concept. However, Goolishian, Anderson, Pullman, and Winderman (1985) have challenged the concept of family by arguing that the problem should be an organizing principle. What this means is that the particular problem should control the decision about who should come to therapy.

Governmental programs shape our data and concepts of families. The Norwegian Census, for example, tends to define family as the household (Befolkningsstatistikken 1988 [1989]), with each person having a *family* number. However, if the person is 18 years or older, married or divorced, he or she is not in the same family as the mother or father who live in the same household. Thus, according to the Norwegian Census, if I had lived in the same household as my mother, we would be considered as two families, each consisting of one person. The difference between Broderick's (1987) position and the Norwegian census is that Broderick sees family as a group and thus consisting of at least two persons. For Broderick, family can be a three-generational unit, which is not possible in the Norwegian census.

A third perspective for defining family can be to see it not only as an institution, but also as the result of the individual's own experiences. This is a perspective of family as a processual concept and not THE family as in the two previous perspectives. Boss (1987), for example, defines family as those whom the person defines as family, a unity that has a past and a future together. Moreover, Jorgenson (1986) operationalizes the idea concerning the individual's definition about who newlyweds with children consider to be their family. Trost, in his article in this volume, suggests that family be defined in terms of dyads. Such a conception means that two persons, either a couple or parent-child unit, may form a family, with any change leading to family re-formations. Through such ideas, different types of families tend not be stereotyped as deviant and hyphen-families get the status of being "real" families.

One problem with having even three different perspectives for understanding definitions of a particular social phenomenon, is that definitions easily become norms. What theoreticians often have meant to be only descriptive, more or less objective and tentative, often becomes normative, even though this was not the original intention. A definition describing how things are easily becomes an expression of what is natural. Definitions may narrow down a phenomenon to an extent that what is outside the definition becomes defined as unnatural or deviant. Although the aim of researchers may not be to specify what is normative, their efforts to reach a unified report relating what "usually" happens may, in the end, help to create a normative outcome.

These three perspectives are not simply a matter of preference, even though the method to be featured here is from the third perspective. Neither are they mutually exclusive. For different purposes various definitions can be useful. One way is to view them as in communication or in relation to each other. For example, the census tells us about variations and changes in household structures. By comparing the census with theoretical definitions, one may discover if any of the normative definitions really are found in the general population in large numbers. Thus, although 1990 statistics in Norway indicate that a quarter of all marriages are remarriages, according to normative definitions, these marriages will not be recognized, despite their prevalence in large numbers. Instead, if we use the individual's empirical experience as a primary base, we could provide important feed-back to the other "normative" perspectives. As it currently stands, however, when individuals experience discrepancies between their own family and the official definition of family, the traditional way is for the person to define the difference as being deviant or somehow their fault.

Although preferable for scholars to have some consensus, as lay persons, we do not need to agree on what a family is in general or of what our own family consists. From an outside perspective, we can never determine what a family is for a specific person. Instead, we can know relatively easily the members of a household, but not the family. Many colleagues who contribute to the family literature, however, seem to "know" what family is or should be. For example, Furstenberg (1987) uses such terms as "omit," "fail" or "exclude" when informants did not count as family members those that Furstenberg "knew" were members. Similarly, Ihinger-Tallman and Pasley (1987) state that a non-residential child, who was not defined as a family member by the interviewee, was "forgotten" and "omitted." Such omissions indicate "ambiguous family boundaries," with the omission indicating a weak sense of family identity.

The Background of a Method to Define Family from the Perspective of the Individual

Although everyday agendas do not include thinking about who belongs to a family and the family relationships between members, the conceptualization of family influences a great deal of one's daily life, including whom one contacts and how one behaves towards them. Skolnick (1973) calls this phenomenon "backstage" knowledge.

The proposed method of discovering who is family from the individual's perspective draws on techniques used in family therapy. The family sculpture technique consists of a certain number of wooden pieces in various sizes that are used to symbolize persons belonging to different generations and gender. This technique also includes symbols for pets. A key component of this procedure involves the placement the wooden pieces on a checker board by an informant, so that the distance between the pieces can be assessed.

Kvebaek's sculpture technique is based on the idea that, when the structure of a family is changing, the positions of family members will change as well (Cromwell, Fournier & Kvebaek, 1980). Thus, one could say that when positions change, these changes could have an effect on the structure over time. This variety of family sculpturing strategies was first developed as an aid to therapy, but now is used in research as well.

Jorgenson (1986) examined how newlywed couples with small children define a family from a communication and psychological perspective. She uses person-like pieces of paper without gender differentiation, with each child getting a limited number of figures (fourteen each). When the interview is over, the location that each interviewee had placed each family member is noted.

Jorgenson developed this method specifically for research, but this procedure can also be used in therapy. Jorgenson made Kvebaek's sculpture technique easier to use, but in doing so, she failed to take note of gender. However, because gender is universally important and an organizing principle in relationships, I am hesitant not to differentiate between males and females. Although C. W. Lidz and V. Lidz (1988) emphasize that gender should not be a variable in qualitative research, the use of the concept "human beings" instead of gender seems to obscure various social realities that we need to recognize and understand.

Jorgenson (1986) has been interested in definitions of family, while both Kvebaek (Cromwell, Fournier & Kvebaek, 1980) and Jorgenson focused on family relationships. Both of their methods have been an inspiration for the method presented in this study (Levin 1989b, 1990, 1994). Another source of inspiration has been my work with Marla Isaacs for the Families of Divorce Project, at the Philadelphia Child Guidance Clinic (Isaacs & Levin, 1984). We used circular and triangular pieces of paper in that study to symbolize female and male family members respectively. In contrast to both Jorgenson's and Kvebaek's work, however, the interviewees were given an unlimited number of pieces so that no restriction was placed on the number of people included in a respondent's concept of family.

This method also differs from those of Kvebaek and Jorgenson in that the subject glues the pieces on the sheet when the interview is finished. This is important because it (1) provides a baseline map for the interviewee and (2) enables comparisons of the maps from various time periods, which is useful for longitudinal research, and therapy. This method catches some processes of change and the actors' own perception of such change. The interviewer can ask, "Two years ago you made this map and now it is different. What has happened?"

This method can be used for new family forms, making it open enough to include the whole family system and narrow enough to focus on the specific area of investigation. Using more than one technique allows one to move slowly into the area of interest, create an interest, increase the subject's consciousness through visualizations and then in the interview to explore and explicate the phenomenon.

The Procedure

The method is divided into three steps: *a family list, a family map* and a *verbal interview.* Each step gives important information and can be used alone, but the method as a whole has a greater richness.

> *The Family List.* The interviews start with a question about the informant's experience of family membership or the "family list." The informant is asked: "When you think of your family, who do you think of? Make a list over those you consider to be your family."

The question is asked without any further introduction, in order to get the interviewee's unbiased answer. If the interviewee has questions like "Who shall I include?", the simple answer is, "It's up to you," and the original question is repeated without any reformations. The interviewee writes the names on a sheet of paper and when finished, reads the names or relationships aloud.

In the analysis, the first question of interest is who are actually included, and then what criteria are decisive for membership: relationships or positions? Are there any persons the informant thought of including, but decided not to include? What was decisive for that choice? The list "belongs" to the informant and can be changed at any time during the whole interview. Sometimes the informant thinks of other persons as family members later in the interview, and is free to add or subtract them whenever wanted.

The Family Map. The family list is followed by creating a family map. The interviewee is asked to place each family member symbolized by the pieces of paper, on a large sheet, approximately 20" by 20". No size differences exist in the pieces of paper that symbolize adults or children. The triangles are 1.75" (4 cm) long and the circles have a diameter of 1.5" (3.5 cm) and are the same color.

The instructions are:

- Would you please place your family on this sheet using these pieces of paper? The triangles are males and the circular pieces are women.
- Would you start with yourself and then put the others according to how close or how distant you feel they are to you? The map is supposed to show the situation as it looks to you today.

Frequently, the informants use a considerable amount of time to find exactly where to place each family member. Afterwards, they are asked to glue the pieces on the sheet and to write the names and/or relationships on them. Some might indicate the geographical distance between the family members. If, for example, a parent is living far away, he or she might be placed far away from the interviewee. This can be corrected by instructions to interviewees that a map of the emotional and not geographical distance is desired.

In my study of stepfamilies (Levin, 1994), attention was focused on the individual's perception of his/her family at the time of the interview. An individual's more general perception of family can be assessed more accurately with the instruction that "independent of how you feel right now, I want you to make a map of the way you usually think of the situation."

The Verbal Interview. The verbal interview is conducted as the last part of the method. The interviewee is given an opportunity to explain what and why the pieces were placed where they were. The interviewee will then be given the possibility of giving more information than the map shows. The verbal interview, together with the map and the list, provides a "triangulation" of the method.

This method provides a means to assess an individual's perception of what or whom constitutes a family at the time of the study and the nature of the relationships between himself or herself and the identified family members. The map is a snapshot and a representation of the individual's perception of the given situation. It does not attempt to provide an objective map of the real situation, but is how the individual perceives it. What is the truth for the individual! If the study were repeated the day after and the result was different, it would not necessarily be a sign of an unreliable method or instrument. This method assumes that human life is a process, with constant change occurring as a part of a process that will define a family.

CONCLUSION

Although many scientific discussions have dealt with defining THE family, a method is presented in this article that is intended to assess the persons that (1) an individual includes in his or her family, (2) how the individual perceives his or her relationships with those family members, and (3) how emotionally close or distant are the members. Historically the method is related to Moreno's (1934) ideas, but differs clearly from his sociometrical methods that are primarily used to clarify the individual's wish for contacts. Because this method examines the perceived distance and membership in various groups, it also differs from other network methods that seek to clarify the frequency of contacts with other persons.

The method was developed to study step families, but can be used for a variety of families and for other groups characterized by close relationships. Who is a friend of whom? Who is a pal of whom? Who feels closeness to whom? Bolstad (1995) used this method in Norway to examine whether parents who gave up their children unwillingly to foster-care, still included their children within their families. Horneman (1996) has used the method to get former clients to make lists and later maps of those who helped them when they were clients. Overall, this method has received positive responses in research since it was first introduced and presented.

This method is not a finished product and it remains to be seen what conclusions can be drawn about many issues. For instance, it is still unclear how the three parts of the method–the family list, the family map, and the verbal interview–overlap or complement each other. Will the map show the same phenomena as what is assessed in the verbal interview? Or, does the map give a different picture? Moreover, it remains to be seen if the list, the map, and the verbal interview assess the same phenomenon or phenomena in different studies. For example, will a long distance placement on the map be an indication of distance in the interviewee's perception of his or her social reality?

To establish contact in research is connected with certain types of challenges without influencing data. The method is especially aimed at providing a simple and relatively rapid way of moving into an emotionally complicated area. A combination of techniques seems to be especially useful for assessing emotionally complicated material. Inner images are caught by visual transformation on a sheet of paper. The construction of the map by itself is a process through which the client is challenged to think about his or her relationships to the family and family members. Before one puts down the pieces, one will reflect upon where the piece should be placed in terms of the question "How close is that person to me?" The task by itself is a way of distancing oneself–it is not the daughter who is placed on the sheet, but the piece that symbolizes her. This can help to get contact with and talk about emotionally complicated matters more easily than dealing with the real circumstances. This task is very close to the person's reality, but, at the same time, provides distance so that family issues can be engaged quickly.

Although this method does not replace family sculpture, it can be used in therapy when the therapist does not know who and/or what a family is defined as. When the perception is changing about who family members are, the therapist can avoid being moralistic by striving to make the client fit a certain type of family or a concept decided upon in advance. The method challenges therapists to view reality from the client's perspective and thus to a dynamic not a static or normative concept of family. Consequently, the possibilities for deeper understanding will be enhanced and the potential for intervention will become more realistic, i.e., more in concordance with the social reality in which the client lives.

Finally, the method may assist in the educational process about the family or other small groups (Levin & Trost, 1992). To teach about family can be difficult simply because the content of the term *family* varies from person to person as well as in time and space. To lecture about this problem does not give the same type of insight as if one uses the method presented here as an exercise for the students.

An important strength of this method is the ability to open up emotional material in a fairly rapid manner. Although an advantage in both therapy and research, this can be dangerous in education and caution should be used. When using this method as an exercise with a particular student, the other students will be able to hear what is said. One has to evaluate in every specific situation, therefore, if the family map, or the family interview, or just the family list should be used. The communication between teacher and the student in explaining what the map means, has to be properly reflected upon in advance, and appropriate referrals to more in-depth treatment need to be available.

A non-problematicized concept of family allows certain types of interpretations of social reality to arise. The more that use is made of complex and less normative concepts, the better will be our interpretations of social reality and the real life circumstances of individuals. The concepts we use help to decide what we can see and what actions we are able to take.

REFERENCES

Befolkningsstatistikken 1988 (1989). *hefte III*, SSB, Oslo.

Bell, N. W., & Vogel, E. F. (1960). Introductory essay: Toward a framework for functional analysis of family behavior. In N. W. Bell & E. F. Vogel (Eds.), *A modern introduction to the family*. Glencoe, IL: Free Press.

Bolstad, T. (1995). Fra moedrenes synsvinkel (From the perspective of the mothers), *Social Work Reports, 17*.

Boss, P. (1987). In an educational tape coordinated by Bert Adams: What is family? Annenberg School of Communication, CPB course on family.

Broderick, C. (1987). In an educational tape coordinated by Bert Adams: What is family? Annenberg School of Communication, CPB course on family.

Caplow, T., Bahr, H. M., Chadwick, B. A., Hill, R., & Williamson, M. H. (1982). *Middletown families: Fifty years of change and continuity.* Minneapolis: University of Minnesota Press.

Cromwell, R., Fournier, D. & Kvebaek, D. (1980). *The Kvebaek family sculpture technique: A diagnostic and research tool in family therapy.* Jonesboro, Tennessee: Pilgrimage.

Furstenberg, F. F. Jr. (1987). The new extended family: The experience of parents and children after remarriage. In K. Pasley & M. Ihinger-Tallman (Eds.), *Remarriage & stepparenting: Current research and theory.* NY: Guildford Press.

Goolishian, H., Anderson, H., Pullman, G., & Winderman, L. (1985). The Galveston Family Institute: Some personal and historical perspectives. Galveston, Texas: Stensil Galveston Family Institute.

Gross, P. (1987). Defining post-divorce remarriage families: A typology based on the subjective perceptions of children. *Journal of Divorce, 10,* 205-217.

Gubrium, J. F., & Holstein, J. A. (1990). *What is family?* Mountain View, CA: Mayfield Publishing Company.

Horneman, K. (1996). *Relasjonen ungdom-hjelper, en studie av ungdom som har vaert i hjelpeapparatets moete med hjelpere (The relationship between youth and helper).* Unpublished master thesis, Program for sosialt arbeid, Universitetet i Trondheim.

Ihinger-Tallman, M., & Pasley, K. (1987). *Remarriage.* Newbury Park, CA: Sage Publications.

Isaacs, M. B., & Levin, I. R. (1984). Who's in my family? A longitudinal study of children of divorce. *Journal of Divorce, 7*(4), 1-21.

Jorgenson, J. (1986). *The family's construction of the concept of 'family.'* Unpublished doctoral dissertation. University of Pennsylvania, Philadelphia.

Levin, I. (1989a). Barnetegninger-stefamiliens fingeravtrykk? (Children drawings-the fingerprint of the stepfamily?) In I. R. Levin & G. Clifford (Eds.), *Relasjoner (Relationships): Hverdagsskrift until Per Olav Tiller.* Trondheim: Tapir.

Levin, I. (1989b). Familie-hva er det? (Family-what is that?). En presentasjon av en metode. *Fokus paa familien, 17,* 25-31.

Levin, I. (1990). How to define family? *Family Reports, 17.* Uppsala University.

Levin, I. (1994). *Stefamilien-Variasjon og mangfold.* Oslo: Aventura.

Levin, I., & Trost, J. (1992). Understanding the concept of family. *Family Relations, 41,* 348-361.

Lidz, C. W., & Lidz, V. (1988). Editors' Note. *Qualitative sociology, 11* (5), 5-7.

Moreno, J. L. (1934). Who shall survive: A new approach to the problem of human interrelations. Washington, DC: Nervous and Mental Disease Publishing Co.

Murdock, G. P. (1949). *Social structure.* Glencoe, IL: The Free Press.

Parsons, T. (1955). *The American family: Its relations to personality and the social structure, Family socialization and interaction process.* Glencoe, IL: The Free Press.

Reiss, I. (1987). In an educational tape coordinated by Bert Adams: What is family? Annenberg School of Communication, CPB course on family.

Rommetveit, R. (1979). On negative rationalism in scholarly studies of verbal communication and dynamic residuals in the construction of human intersubjectivity.

In R. Rommetveit & R. M. Blakar (Eds), *Studies of language, thought and verbal communication*. London: Academic Press.

Settles, B. H. (1987). A perspective on tomorrow's families. In M. B. Sussman & S. K. Steinmetz (Eds.), *Handbook of marriage and the family* (pp. 157-180). NY: Plenum.

Skolnick, (1973). *The intimate environment: Exploring marriage and the family.* Boston: Little, Brown and Company.

Winch, R. F. (1971). *The modern family.* NY: Holt, Rinehart & Winston.

What Are Families After Divorce?

Kari Moxnes

INTRODUCTION

This family, which in the beginning is the only existent social relation, becomes as growing needs create new societal relationships and the growing population creates new needs, a subordinate relationship (except in Germany) and must therefore be dealt with and developed in accordance with the existing empirical data, not with the concept "the family" . . . . (Marx, 1970, page 69, my translation from the Norwegian translation)

In considering the topic "Is there a family after divorce?", I had to consider if what I was asking was whether divorce is the end of the family? A very common assumption is that divorce breaks the family and leaves it in ruins that can no longer be called *'family.'* Is it better to view divorce as a transitional phase in the family career, one that does not end the family, only transforms it into binuclear, single parent, or stepfamilies? My position is that divorce and remarriage, as process, do not necessarily lead to the end of the family, but they do always change a family dramatically (Moxnes, 1984, 1990, 1992b).

An empirical question that will be indirectly addressed in this article is whether families after divorce ought to be called *'families,'* and to what degree are they similar to families before divorce. Another way of understanding the question is more philosophic, as a question of what is that entity

Kari Moxnes is affiliated with the Department of Sociology, University of Trondheim, Dragvoll, Norway.

This article is based on a paper presented at the XXVI International CFR seminar, Norway, 1991.

[Haworth co-indexing entry note]: "What Are Families After Divorce?" Moxnes, Kari. Co-published simultaneously in *Marriage & Family Review* (The Haworth Press, Inc.) Vol. 28, No. 3/4, 1999, pp. 105-120; and: *Concepts and Definitions of Family for the 21st Century* (ed: Barbara H. Settles et al.) The Haworth Press, Inc., 1999, pp. 105-120. Single or multiple copies of this article are available for a fee from The Haworth Document Delivery Service [1-800-342-9678, 9:00 a.m. - 5:00 p.m. (EST). E-mail address: getinfo@haworthpressinc.com].

or the social phenomenon that we call family after the divorce. This will be addressed, not so much by way of a philosophic discussion of what families really are, but by discussing how family sociologists might get a better understanding of families, regardless of whether the "objects" of inquiry are families before divorce, after divorce, or after remarriage.

According to my point of view, as long as people, you and I, think, talk and act as if there is something existing that we call families, they exist, not as an object or a concrete thing, but as a social construction. It is these social constructions, and the continuous social construction processes, that constitute our field of inquiry. This article is about how we can study these social constructions. At the same time it is a criticism of definitional family studies. Finally it is an illustration of the approach I have chosen and used when studying families.

In the first part of this paper, I will present my position that because the concept of '*the family*' is to a large degree is an ideological idea, it is of no value as a scientific concept. When studying families we have to deconstruct them by studying the different ideological and material structures and processes that constitute families and the relationships between families. Next, I will provide an illustration of the limitations of "definitional" family research, showing the necessity of deconstructing the families. In this part I will use my own family as an example.

IDEOLOGICAL FAMILY DEFINITIONS: THE FAMILY

In everyday conversation, in mass media, and in sociological studies, the concept of "THE FAMILY" is frequently used. The family, written large, makes it appear that there is only one family, that the family is a concrete thing, a natural entity, universal and ahistorical (Moxnes-Osmundsen, 1979). Furthermore, using the concept in such a way gives the impression that everybody knows what the family is, and that the meaning and valuation of the concept is the same for everyone.

You have only to ask a few people what they think of when hearing the word '*family*,' and you might get as many different answers as the number of people you have asked. Some will tell you about their family of origin, others of their single-parent family, while others talk about their reconstructed family. When people "talk" family, they use two different concepts. The first, "THE FAMILY," is an ideological concept. The second is the concept people use when referring to what they see as empirical families.

"*The family*" is an ideological concept because it is an ideal; being family, having family, and living in a happy family is what most of us want and think is necessary to have a happy life. It is not a false ideal. In our society where the family has almost a monopoly on close human relations, intimacy and happiness, it is no wonder that people look to the family for such relations. Furthermore, the family is ideology because it is used as a political concept. It is the traditional patriarchal family that is presented as the ideal. Finally the family is ideology, meaning false consciousness because it is "a cover up," giving a false picture of what families really are (Barrett & McIntosh, 1982; Thorne & Yalom, 1982; Moxnes, 1981, 1990).

"*The family*" is the romantic story of boy meeting girl, getting married, having children, making a home, and living happily ever after. It is the family based on romantic, erotic love, glued together by the promise of lifelong love and exclusive sexuality, formalized by marriage, and fulfilled by having children and setting up a home. It is a unit made of emotional, legal and biological bonds. It is also the family that Parsons (1965) described and considered to be ideal: the family with a male head, the instrumental father, the breadwinner, and the dependent wife, mother, and housekeeper. It is the private family, the closed-off world where women and children often are beaten and sexually abused. Under these circumstances it becomes a male "haven in a heartless world" (Lasch, 1977). From a feminist point of view "*the family*" is a patriarchal concept that has played an important part in securing male domination over women, and control of the women and children in the family (Liljestrom, 1983).

"*The family*" is also the basis of our definition of family; a family where the couple are legally married and are the biological parents of one or more children. They are seen as units because they have the "right" combination of "glue"; legal, biological and supposedly emotional "glue." Families that lack one or more of the "glue components" are considered to be neither reliable units nor real families. Married couples without children are not real families, but they might become that. Couples who are not married, but cohabit and live under marriage-like conditions are not real families. They lack the "glue" of the marriage license. However, they might be considered to be a real family in time, when they have become parents and have stayed together for a number of years.

The Single-Parent Family

Even though all single-parent families are considered to be deviant, the female-headed single-parent families, which are in the majority, are seen as worse than the male-headed families. The family of the divorced mother is considered to be the second most deviant family because she who has left her husband (as you know, most divorces are initiated by the woman). However, the least acceptable single-parent family is the family of the never-married mother, the one in which the woman has managed the entire time without a man. The most accepted single-parent family is the family of the divorced father; such families are seen as somewhat heroic.

Family concepts are, of course, also social products. At the same time as the negative concept of "the single-parent family" is frequently in use, a new and different concept of "the after-divorce family" is being constructed. According to this concept, divorce is not the end of the family, divorce is only the end of the marriage, of the spousal relationship. After the divorce the nuclear family becomes an extended family including old and new family members. The parental relationship continues and the spousal relationship is turned into friendship. This concept is an ideal, but it is also ideology because it gives a false picture of reality. Since there is no empirical study showing that this is a common family career after divorce (Ahrons & Rodgers, 1987; Moxnes, 1990), there is no reason to believe that any large number of parents share parenthood equally after divorce, or become good friends.

The Step Family

If divorce is regarded as bad and as the end of the family, remarriage is considered to be good and to be the only way of mending a broken or ruined family. It is the only way of making a family whole again, or of including the 'familyless' into the sanctuary of families. Even though there are negative connotations associated with the concept, "the stepfamily," stepfamilies are seen as better than not having a family or living in a single-parent family.

In everyday social exchange, it is usually no great communication problem when the ideological concept of family and the more empirically oriented concept of family are substituted for each other. In such situations we usually know the context, the embeddedness of what is said. However in other situations it is hard to differentiate between the two concepts. It may be the goal of the substitution is to conceal the difference between ideal and reality, as when presenting our own family life as almost identical to the ideal.

An important reason for concealing the difference between ideal and reality is that families are important to us. Family life is a main part of our lives, we are families, have families, and live in families. We do not distinguish between these two concepts because "the family" is ideology, the ideal that we want to believe that our own and most other families are examples of. Therefore, many researchers as well as the general public prefer to believe in the concept of "the family" instead of acknowledging the often grim reality of real family life. That, I believe, is one of the reasons why so many family sociologists have done research on and by means of ideological family definitions, instead of studying the social phenomenon that we call families.

STUDYING FAMILIES BY MEANS OF DEFINITIONS

When doing sociological work one should not, as Marx correctly stated years ago, let an ideological concept, *"the family,"* be what we are studying.

What we ought, but often only pretend, to study are the social constructions that come in a myriad of shapes and colors that we call families. Too many sociologists have been studying family definitions instead of families. The most common form of such misuse is when *"the family"* is used as a model or the yardstick to which all kinds of families are compared or measured against. When comparing empirical families to an ideological definition, most families–whether they are called nuclear, single-parent or step-families, dual earner or traditional complementarian, loving or violent families–come out looking deviant and lacking something essential. This is what Ganong and Coleman (1987) call a "deficit comparison model." This is amply illustrated in textbooks in family sociology, or the *Handbook of Marriage and the Family* (Sussman & Steinmetz, 1986) where the reader can find a large number of studies referred to that use the concept of the family as described above.

When we study families by means of definitions, we are not studying "families," but rather are studying measurement, the definition, and the degree one's measurement fits the empirical families under study. To study families, we need to find out how people define family and how they live their family-lives, not to decide beforehand what families are. If families had been a thing, a unit, natural, universal and ahistoric, then we could have searched for "the essence of family," or for all the little bits and parts that together make family. We all acknowledge, when doing research, that families are not a thing or a concrete object, that it is futile to search for the essence of family, and that families are neither universal nor ahistorical.

Even though we can find something that resembles what we call families in all known cultures, we know from Ira Reiss (1971) that a universal definition of the family cannot be a useful scientific concept and is of little help in understanding what families are. The most precise definition he could make was the following: "The family institution is a small kinship structured group with the key function of nurturant socialization" (Reiss, 1971:19). We also know that a family is not necessarily a unit. As Leena Alanen (1986:4) correctly states:

> The proper object of a sociology of families is to be found 'behind' the taken-for-granted unity of 'the family' and if [there is] unity . . . , this unity should be a problem needing explanation, not a fact to be assumed.

STUDYING FAMILIES AS SOCIAL CONSTRUCTIONS

Families are social constructions, products of a given society's way of organizing its members' sexuality (Liljestrom, 1983), the social differentiation of the society and its economic and production systems (Shorter, 1976; Gaunt, 1983; Goody, 1983; Anderson, 1980). Because families are social products, they must be studied in their historical, cultural, ethical and class variability. Because families are social constructions, it is necessary to deconstruct them to understand what families are. Mitchell (1973), who saw that *"the family"* was an ideological construct, recommended a destructuralization of the family. Only by studying the functions; reproduction, production, sexuality and socialization that together are the basis of families, can we disclose the reality of families.

Barrett and McIntosh (1982) recommended the deconstruction of the family, saying that we have to disclose the falseness of our understanding of what families are, at the same time as we show how families, kinship systems, households, the sexual division of work, and family ideologies are social products. As sociologists we must study the variability in ideological and material structures and processes that together constitute families and the relationship between families. Liljestrom (1980) emphasizes the importance of differentiating between family forms and the family as a social-psychological group, while Rapp (1982) advises us to differentiate between families and households and to study the relationships between the two. Gullestad (1984) underlines the importance of differentiating between family and household, or 'team' and 'task,' and recommends that the household be studied as a moral community. By focusing on the relations, the analysis of family and household gets tied together.

This means that we ought to study *"the family"* as ideology, as defined and lived by family members, as a system of relationships with biological and emotional ties, and as households. No matter what we call the families we are studying, nuclear, single parent, or reconstructed families, we have to deconstruct them in order to understand what families are, how they function and how they develop and change. Studying divorced or reconstructed families is no different from studying nuclear families, but it is often more complicated because of the greater variety of family patterns, relationships between family members and organization of the household. When studying families after divorce, the importance of differentiating between family and household is obvious.

When families are viewed as social constructions, such an understanding has important implications for how we can conduct our research. We have to go to the social constructors themselves to find out what these social constructions are and how they are constructed and reconstructed. Based on the information, the facts, concepts and cultural categories we get from the social actors, we have to make our own description, what Schutz (1967) calls *"the construct of first degree."* Based on these descriptions and using all the theoretical tools sociologists have, we need to analyze, search for analytic categories, and make our *"construct of second degree"* (Schutz, 1967) that ought to give us all a better understanding of what families are, and how they change.

STUDYING MY FAMILY

Even though most books on scientific methods recommend that the scientist be an objective distant observer, I have decided to let the ever-changing social construction that I call my family be the one and only example when trying to illustrate the shortcomings of traditional family studies and the necessity of deconstruction in order to understand the very complex social phenomenon called family. I do this because years of studying other people's families has taught me that deep inside knowledge is important especially when trying to understand what families are.

My Family Before Divorce

Fifteen years ago, I would have told you that my family consisted of my husband, my son, my daughter and myself. An ordinary family. At that time my husband was the only income earner in the family, and most people considered me to be a housewife. A common way of sharing family responsibilities at that time. Our relationship was as it ought to be, based on romantic love. My husband and I met in the Student Union in Trondheim in 1964. (Getting a husband with a degree from the Norwegian Institute of Technology was what most girls from this town hoped for.) After having been sweethearts for a couple of years we got engaged. One year later, in 1968 we married in the church and had a lovely wedding. Everything was properly done. After a few years there were four of us, my husband, my two children, and me living in a single-family house in the forest on the outskirts of Trondheim.

If a sociologist equipped with a ready-made definition of the family–the nuclear family–had come to study (measure) my family at that time, he would have found a family that on the surface resembled the definition to a large degree. We must have looked like the perfect family. Four people living in a little red house in the forest–the peaceful and healthy Norwegian way of living. Two well-behaved, very blond children, the oldest a boy, the youngest a girl–exactly what most parents want. The husband a successful engineer in programming, who earned a good salary, and me, the wife, a good and efficient housekeeper, who made most of her own and the children's clothes.

From an ideological point of view this was "the family," a unit, just the way such units are supposed to be. From a statistical point of view this was the normal family, the average family of the time. Studied as a household this family would also have come out as average. The household size and the standard of living were average, and the sharing of household tasks (I have to confess) had over the years become more and more traditional.

However, when using a ready-made definition to study families you can only measure those factors that the measurement is made to measure and only see to what degree the "object" under study fits the definition. The public image of my family at that time did fit the definition perfectly. The private image, however, was quite different, but the sociologist studying my family could not detect that using his kind of measurement; the definition of the nuclear family. He could not discover that the traditional way of sharing household tasks had become a major problem, and that the unity of the family was nothing but appearance. I, the mother, had reluctantly had to realize that the only unit that existed in the family consisted of the children and me. The father had, as frequently happens with fathers, become a peripheral person in the family (Monsen, 1975). The spousal relationship had become one of frustration and anger, there was little parental cooperation, since most of the work with the children was left to the mother, and the father-child relationships were emotionally distant. What the sociologist could have done to detect such important aspects of this family's life, I will return to later when discussing my after-divorce family.

Ten years ago my husband and I separated, and later divorced. The important question concerning the divorce is not, as I have stated earlier, whether the divorce was the end of the family, or if the divorce led to single-parent or remarried families, but how a sociologist best can study the process of change and the great variety of results of divorce, how they can study the social construction that divorced people call family.

My Family After Divorce

After the divorce I continued to live in the little red house with my children. Years before the divorce I had finished my studies and found work at the University. I was able to support the children and myself fairly well. An outsider, a neighbor, observing our family from such a perspective might have been surprised to find no major changes except the fact that the children's father no longer lived with us. Being a family member, things looked quite different. The children and I went through radical changes. We had to change our understanding of what a family is, change the relationships between us, and find new ways of organizing our household. From the point of view of a traditional sociologist, however, we had gone through dramatic changes, we had stopped being a family or become a deviant family.

Measured by Definition

Using the definition of "the family" to study or measure my family after divorce is meaningless; such an enterprise could only lead to the conclusion that my family was very deviant or was not a family at all. Studying my "after-divorce family" by using the traditional very negative definition of "the single-parent family" that I have earlier described, would not provide much information either. Measured by that definition my family would again come out as deviant. Except for the very first months after the separation, my "after-divorce family" has been a happy, well-functioning family. I have earned a good salary and the children's father has paid a substantial amount of money in support of his children. We have never lived in poverty. My children have not been noticeably damaged by growing up in a single-parent family. They did not lose their father; on the contrary, they developed a better relationship with him after the divorce.

On the other hand, my "after-divorce family" does not really resemble the new positive definition of the single-parent family as part of the binuclear family. Even if my children think of their family as a binuclear family consisting of two households (Ahrons, 1979), my own after-divorce family is not an extended family that includes my former husband, neither do I regard him to be a friend.

Shortly after my divorce I met a man who became my lover. Since he was also a single parent living with his two sons, we decided that we could not marry or live together. We both knew that forcing four teenagers to live together in one home was too much to ask of them. We also knew that such an arrangement could have ruined the loving relationship between us in a matter of weeks. However, after seven years of living alone with my children, I sold my house and bought half of my lover's house.

Comparing my after-divorce family to the definition of stepfamily does not work either. Even if my partner and I now live in the same house and share the same bed, there is not much else that resembles a stepfamily. Since using ready-made ideological definition to study my family in different stages in my life is insufficient, and gives little information, one ought to try other approaches.

Studied as a Household

Families are frequently studied as households–two concepts that frequently are not differentiated. If a sociologist came to study the household I live in today, he or she would probably bring with him a questionnaire based on what is considered common knowledge regarding households in Norway. The sociologist might begin by asking about the number of people living in the household. My response to that question would be, "7 or 4 people, depending on how a household is defined." If where you sleep is an indicator of household, my household contains seven people. If where you eat is the main indicator, I live in a household of four people most of the week, and of seven people on weekends. If I were to show the sociologist my house, he or she would see that in my apartment or flat, there are three bedrooms, one for each of my three grown children. Furthermore he would see that in my lover's flat there are also three bedrooms: one for each of his grown children, and one that he and I share.

At this stage in the interview, the sociologist, as a good scientist, would really get interested. The sociologist would now have to ask if what was being studied was one household or two households. Using common indicators the sociologist would inquire about the ownership of the house and the apartments, and how the house was used. I would tell this person that we owned the house together, that everything concerning the house was equally shared, both financially and in regards to household upkeep and maintenance. However, one of the four flats or apartments in the house is mine and one other is called his. My children and I spend most time in our flat, but over the last few years, we are frequently using the two flats as if they were one home. If a visitor is coming, or if we are having a party we use the apartment that is free or the one that has been cleaned recently.

The sociologist would probably have trouble deciding whether this should be regarded as one household or two households. If the sociologist insisted on using the standard questionnaire it would probably not have a category for a household such as ours. The sociologist would have to make a choice, either register us as one household or as two separate households. This choice would result in some very important information being lost, as well as the possibility to learn something new about households. We are not living in one or two households, but all of us live concurrently in two households.

If the sociologist continued to ask about the sharing of the daily household tasks, the sociologist would find that both my lover and I are breadwinners, that we have developed a very complicated economic system of both private and shared economy. Asking about the sharing of other household tasks one might get answers that were not expected, answers for which there is no place on the questionnaire to register. The answers might be unexpected because in this household the mother and the father are not the main housekeepers. We very seldom do household tasks, even though we are the administrators of the household. All cleaning, and most of the cooking, is left to the children who take turns and get paid to do this work. Such a way of sharing household tasks is not common in nuclear families; but it is common in single-parent households with older children.

Shortly after divorce, most single parents try to be both mother and father for their children, and to do all the work themselves that two parents used to do. However, after a while, the workload becomes too heavy, and new ways of organizing the household are developed. Often, and especially if the head of the household plans to stay single for a while, the result is an organization where the children take a substantial part of the household work and responsibility (Moxnes, 1990, 1992a, 1992b). Who is doing the work has been the determining factor in the organization of our household. The household might be seen as organized in two different ways. Most of the week we behave as if we are two households. That means that we eat separately. On weekends, however, we behave as if we are one household.

Continuing to respond to questions about the relationship between the household members, I would tell the sociologist that my apartment is occupied by my biological son (21 years old), and daughter (19 years old), my social daughter (19 years old), and myself. My social daughter is a student from Australia, living with us for a year as part of our family. In the other flat lives my lover and my two social sons, 20 and 19 years old. I doubt very much that there would be categories on the questionnaire that fitted all the different relationships in our household. The sociologist would have to register this as one male-headed, single-parent household with two grown children and one female-headed household with three grown children. This would then overlook the fact that my social daughter is not mine in the biological sense; the sociologist could register us as mother with two grown children and one person living in the household, not belonging to the family. That option again misses some important information regarding my relationship with my social daughter.

If our sociologist really wanted to understand our household he or she would not try to fit us into a precoded questionnaire. Instead the sociologist would ask us and try to understand: (a) How we define our household, (b) How we organize our household, and (c) Why we have chosen to live in such a household. Using this data one would then get the facts we give to him or her and the cultural categories we use. The sociologist could make his or her descriptions, and develop his or her "construct of first degree" (Schutz, 1967).

Studied as Defined by Family Member

By now I hope that our sociologist has given up trying to fit my household and family into a common category, or to measure us by way of ideological definitions. The person has finally understood that I, as well as all others, are social constructors who make our own definitions of family, just as we develop and change our family lives. The only way of getting the information we need to understand and explain what my family is, is by using the approach recommended above by asking people–the other family members and me: What is family? who do you consider to be family? and why do you consider them to be family members?

Since my research in 1984 as well as in a number of studies, I have used a family drawing as a source of data. Before interviewing adults and children, the participants are asked to draw a picture which includes all the members that they consider to belong to their family. After they have completed their drawing, I ask them to tell me who these people are and provide them with the opportunity to indicate if there is someone else that they had thought of, but decided not to include in the drawing. Next I ask why those in the picture were included, and why others were not. When these questions have been answered, I will know why some are considered to be family members while others are not. Finally, I ask about the relations between all the members of the family, especially the closeness and emotional bonds between them. This is the technique that Levin (Levin, 1990; Levin & Trost, 1992) later developed into a methodology for gathering data. If our sociologist had asked all the members of my household these questions, the first thing that would be noticed was that all of us would draw different family pictures. Some will draw a picture including only a few people, others one with many people, but none of the pictures would have included the very same people.

I will not describe all the family pictures the members of my household drew when I was preparing this article, but will describe my picture as well as those of my biological son and daughter to illustrate the value of this exercise. In my drawing of the family, I place myself in the center. Close to me are my biological son and daughter and my lover; a little further away is my social daughter, my two social sons and my mother and father. Extending the family outside the household I include one aunt who is very dear to me, my brother and his family, and my social parents in the United States.

My daughter's picture included the whole of our household, her father's household, my parents, and her grandparents. My son's picture was much smaller; he had only included his father, his sister and me. My lover's and my social children's pictures were of course different, they included a former spouse, and their biological mother and father.

Some might dislike that I include social sons, daughters and parents in my family picture, because they believe or prefer terms like mother, father, son, daughter, brother and sister to be reserved for those who are biologically, or at least legally related. I disagree with such a view. The limitations in studying families by means of definition also apply to studies of family relations. Insisting on biological and/or legal definitions of family relations excludes studies of important aspects of family life, namely how people who are not biologically related become family members. These processes are also parts of the social construction of families. This is an important issue in our time because of the high divorce and remarriage rates that make a rapidly increasing number of people become social parents and children. It is therefore necessary to study relationships in households and families as defined by the respondents, since not all members may be biologically related.

Studied as a System of Relations

I will not describe all 21 dyadic relationships in our household, but will limit myself to describing my own relationships to the other family members. My children and I have lived alone for eight years, in that time I am convinced that we have developed relationships that are closer and more egalitarian than most parent-child relationships in two-parent families. My relationships with my son and daughter are mother-child relationships, but also friendships based on trust and respect. If my beliefs are correct, this is in accordance with what I and others have found when studying female-headed, single-parent families (Moxnes, 1990, 1991).

The main reasons for the closeness and the egalitarianism that are often found in single-parent families are because the children actively participate in household activities, and single parents often use their older children as confidantes and friends. In such households the interdependency between parent and children becomes so obvious that it cannot be ignored, since as a consequence more democratic or egalitarian relationships are developed.

My relationship with my social daughter from Australia developed rapidly. When she arrived almost a year ago, I did not know her. Now I feel as if she is mine, my daughter. I recognize that my feelings for her are different from my feelings for my biological children, but that is partly because I have had a much longer history with them. My feelings for my social daughter are also different from and much more motherly than my feelings for other children, such as my brother's children who are very dear to me. My social daughter and I have developed a mother-child relationship because we have behaved like a mother and a daughter towards each other. Feeling like a mother comes from behaving like a mother. You might think that I am exaggerating, that it is impossible or unusual to develop such a relationship with a 19-year-old child in a matter of months, but I have experienced it the other way around. In 1962-1963, I was an exchange student in Oklahoma. Ever since then, I have emotionally had two sets of parents. Mom and Dad in the States are also my parents.

My relationships with my two social sons are different. When I got to know those two boys years ago, I consciously avoided becoming any kind of mother-figure for them. I insisted on being only their father's lover and hopefully a good adult friend to them. Being a mother means being responsible, and I thought I had enough being mother to my own children. I also told myself that they had a perfectly good mother of their own, even if she was living far away, and even if I did see that on occasions they might need some motherly help and care. As time passed, our relationships changed. I still don't feel like a mother for them, but at times I do motherly tasks, mostly in order to help their father. Even if we have not developed any kind of mother-child relationships, they are definitely part of my family, and an important part of my daily life. I am fond of them, happy with them and proud of them when they succeed, and sad and worried when things are not going their way.

My relationship with my partner is that of a lover and friend relationship. It is like a spousal relationship in that it is monogamous and intended to be lifelong. But we do not have a marriage license. In my opinion our relationship is more egalitarian than most spousal relationships, mostly because there is no dependency between us except emotional dependency. We make an effort trying to be only friends and lovers, not husband and wife in the legal or household sense of these terms. At the same time we have become co-parents in a way, which means that at times we help each other with our grown children, mostly by discussing our worries, or by giving practical help, similar to the stepparent role.

Studied as a Process

After examining my family, which I have defined as a system of relations and as a household, one has quite a lot of information that can provide an understanding of "my family," who is in it, and how it functions. However, you still don't know much about why we have become such a family. To get a holistic understanding of this family, additional information is necessary. Families are not static, they are continuous construction processes. One might call this social construction process 'a family career.' The use of the concept, family career, is not to suggest that there is anything predetermined in the process, nor any predefined stages of development that families go through, as developmental theories often seem to indicate (Hill, 1970; Carter & McGoldrick, 1980). I use the family career concept because it helps focus on two important aspects, continuity and change, in the social construction process.

My family at present is a result of the past, but also of the future. It is the result of, but not the sum of, all the family members' previous family careers, and mainly my lover's and my own hopes for the future. As I see it, I have tried to make a family that is different from the one I had at an earlier stage in my family career. I have some negative experiences from living in a household that became more and more traditional as to the sharing of household tasks.

Therefore, I knew that I would never willingly become someone's wife (meaning subordinate) or housekeeper again. I also knew from having studied remarriage for a number of years that such a family was not what I wanted for myself and for my children. A large number of divorced parents that I had interviewed had convinced me of how difficult living in a step-family household can be, which accounts for the very high divorce rates of second and third marriages. At the same time I knew that my relationship with my lover could be ruined if we did not shorten the distance between our households. Our family, an extended family, our household, a two and one household, and our way of life represent a compromise between having two single-parent households and a step family household. It is also a way of taking care of the love for your partner without having to place too heavy a burden on your children. It is a result of former positive and negative experiences and constructed to give our future together the best possible chances. It is our way of coping, not necessarily the kind of family that I would recommend to others.

CONCLUSIONS

It is time we took Marx's recommendations seriously and stopped studying families by means of definitions. Instead we must use the question, "What is family?" as the guiding light for our research. By deconstructing "*the family*" and by studying the variability in ideologies and material structures and processes that constitute families will we get a better understanding of what families are. By studying the changes in family ideologies, in family compositions, in family relations, and in household organizations we will be able to give better explanations of how families are constructed. To mention a few, we can do as Gubrium and Holstein have done in their book, *What is Family?* (1990), and as others have recommended (Barrett & McIntosh, 1982; Bernardes, in this volume; Thorne & Yalom, 1982) be done. This approach is also valuable for studying divorced families (Ahrons & Rodgers, 1987; Moxnes, 1990). These studies together with a number of others that have used the approach of deconstructing families have brought us a step forward to a better understanding of the social construction called families.

REFERENCES

Ahrons, C. R. (1979). The binuclear family: Two households–one family. *Alternative Life Styles, 2*, 499-515.
Ahrons, C. R., & Rodgers, R. H. (1987). *Divorced Families: A multidisciplinary developmental View.* New York: W. W. Norton & Company.
Alanen, L. (1986). *Socialization and the family: Some theoretical perspectives.* Paper presented at the XI World Congress of Sociology. New Delhi.
Anderson, M. (1980). *Approaches to the history of the western family 1500-1914.* London: Macmillan.
Barrett, M., & McIntosh, M. (1982). *The antisocial family.* London: Verso Editions/NLB.
Carter, E. A., & M. McGoldrick, M. (1980). *The family life cycle: A framework for family therapy.* New York: Gardner Press Inc.
Ganong, L. H., & Coleman, M. (1987). The cultural stereo-typing of stepfamilies. In K. Pasley & M. Ihinger-Tallmann (Eds.), *Remarriage and step-parenting: Current research and theory.* New York: Guilford Press.

Gaunt, D. (1983). *Familieliv i Norden.* Malmo: Gidlunds.

Goody, J. (1983). *The development of the family and marriage in Europe.* Cambridge: Cambridge University.

Gubrium, J. F., & Holstein J. A. (1990). *What is family?* Mountain View, CA: Mayfield Publishing Company.

Gullestad, M. (1984). Sosialantropoligiske perspektiver på familie og hushold. In I. Rudie (Ed.), *Myk start: Hard landing.* Oslo: Universitetsforlaget.

Hill, R. (1970). *Family development in three generations.* Cambridge: Schenkman.

Lasch, C. (1977). *Haven in a heartless world.* New York: Basic Books.

Levin, I. (1990). *How to define family.* Family Reports, No. 17. Uppsala University.

Levin, I., & Trost, J. (1992). Understanding the concept of family. *Family Relations, 41,* 348-361.

Liljestrom, R. (1980). *Uppvekstvilkår.* Uddevalla: Almenna Forlaget.

Liljestrom, R. (1983). *Det erotiska kriget.* Stockholm: Liber Forlag.

Marx, K. (1970). *Verker i utvalg: Skrifter om den materialistiske historieoppfatningen.* Oslo: Pax Forlag.

Mitchell, J. (1973). *Kvinners lodd.* Oslo: Pax Forlag.

Monsen, N. K. (1975). *Det kvinnelige mennesket: Feministisk filosofi.* Oslo: Aschehoug & Co.

Moxnes-Osmundsen, K. (1979). *Ekteskapet: Om ekteskapsproblemer og skilsmisseårsaker.* Magistergrads avh. ISS, Universitetet i Trondheim.

Moxnes, K. (1981). *Når kvinner vil skilles.* Oslo: Pax Forlag.

Moxnes, K. (1984). *Skilt, men fortsatt foreldre.* ISS rapport Nr. 19. ISS, Universitetet i Trondheim.

Moxnes, K. (1990). *Kjernesprengning i familien? Familieforandring ved samlivsbrudd og dannelse av nye samliv.* Doktorgrads avh Universitetsforlaget, Oslo.

Moxnes, K. (1991). Changes in family patterns: Changes in parenting? In U. Bjornberg (Ed.), European parents in the 1990's: Contradictions and change. New Brunswick, NJ: Transaction Publishers.

Moxnes, K. (1992a). One-parent family strategies. In U. Bjornberg (Ed.), *One-parent families in Europe.* Vienna centre.

Moxnes, K. (1992b). *Eneforeldrefamilien som oppvekstmiljo for barn.* NIBR rapport, Oslo.

Parsons, T. (1965). The normal American family. In S. Farber, P. Mustacchi & R. H. L. Wilson (Eds.), *Man and civilization: The family's search for survival.* New York: McGraw Hill.

Rapp, R. (1982). Family and class in contemporary America: Notes toward an understanding of ideology. In B. Thorn & M. Yalom (Eds.), *Rethinking the family.* New York: Longman.

Reiss, I. L. (1971). *The family system in America.* New York: Holt, Rinehart & Winston Inc.

Schutz, A. (1967). *The phenomenology of the social world.* Chicago: Northwestern University Press.

Shorter, E. (1976). *The making of the modern family.* London: Collins.

Sussman, M. B., & Steinmetz, S. K. (Eds.). (1986). *Handbook of marriage and the family.* New York: Plenum Press.

Thorne, B., & Yalom, M. (1982). *Rethinking the family.* New York: Longman.

Trying to Become a Family;
or, Parents Without Children

Ingegerd Wirtberg

INTRODUCTION

The standard medical definition of infertility is: ". . . the inability to achieve a pregnancy after a year of regular sexual relations without the use of contraception, or to carry a pregnancy to live birth" (Meyers, Diamond, Kezur, Scharf, Weinshel & Rait, 1995). In the western world, 15-20% of all couples of child-bearing age–about one couple in six–are affected by infertility (Kraft, Mitchell, Dean, Meyer & Wright-Scmidt, 1980; Lalos, 1985). According to these figures, in the United States there are approximately ten million infertile couples, while in Sweden the total is about one hundred thousand (Lalos, 1985). Infertility has thwarted many couples who desire to have a baby. Not only has infertility prevented them from the prospect of living with biological children, an immediate loss, it also represents the loss of an imagined future (Pengelly, Inglis & Cudmore, 1993).

Dariiluk (1988) suggests that since only about 5% of the world's married population chooses to remain voluntarily childless it appears that becoming a parent continues to be a major life-goal for many men and women. He notes that over the centuries, parenthood has remained a necessary criterion for personal fulfillment, social acceptance, achievement of full adult status, religious membership, sexual identity and psychological adjustment.

Therefore, the concept of the 'childless family' highlights the question, "What is a family?" Trost (1989) found that 75% of his respondents thought that a middle-aged married couple who had no children were a family. How-

Ingegerd Wirtberg is affiliated with the University of Lund, Unit for Postgraduate Psychotherapy Training and Education, Entr. 108, 2nd Floor, S-214 01 Malmö, Sweden.

[Haworth co-indexing entry note]: "Trying to Become a Family; or, Parents Without Children." Wirtberg, Ingegerd. Co-published simultaneously in *Marriage & Family Review* (The Haworth Press, Inc.) Vol. 28, No. 3/4, 1999, pp. 121-133; and: *Concepts and Definitions of Family for the 21st Century* (ed: Barbara H. Settles et al.) The Haworth Press, Inc., 1999, pp. 121-133. Single or multiple copies of this article are available for a fee from The Haworth Document Delivery Service [1-800-342-9678, 9:00 a.m. - 5:00 p.m. (EST). E-mail address: getinfo@haworthpressinc.com].

ever, only 60% thought that a childless couples in their thirties, who had cohabited for three years, were a family. It appears that at least for younger couples, a baby is a requirement for the couple to become a family. When couples had planned their houses, their careers, their economy and their lives in anticipation of becoming parents and the babies did not arrive, the difference between their idea of how they wanted their lives to be, and the way they actually were, created tension, confusion and a strain on their relationships.

The possibility of being infertile, with its attendant loss of parenthood, meant that many couples entered a period of life that was ambiguous, marked by a 'double description' of what reality was and/or could be (Bateson, 1980; Keeney, 1983.) One way of describing these couples is to say that they became 'stuck' in one phase of their life-cycle and were unable to get to the next phase (Carter & McGoldrick, 1988). Their life-style, their expectations, their thoughts and their feelings were all prepared for the transition from a couple to a family–a transition that did not take place.

CHILDLESSNESS IN SWEDEN

To explore the dynamics of involuntary childlessness, a group of 31 couples were followed over a two-year period (Wirtberg, 1992). The couples were selected for the study according to the following criteria: they lived in the same catchment area, they had no children from earlier relationships, and they had turned to the medical system for help with their childlessness.

The importance of children for personal fulfillment, social acceptance, achievement of full adult status, etc., noted earlier by Dariiluk (1988) was affirmed by most of the couples interviewed. For a great majority of these couples (82%), it had always been assumed that they would have children and create a family. Having children was considered to be an integral aspect of the continuity of life and an obvious choice for their future. In response to the question: "Why do you want children?" the most common response was, "It's only natural," or "That is what life is meant for, to have a family and children." Ninety-four percent of women and 84% of men stated that life would be rather pointless if there were no children who could carry on the family's heritage after they died.

Men, but not women, noted this desire for genetic continuity, sometimes expressed as a "dynastic duty" towards their family of origin (Pengelly et al., 1993). However, these men stated that their desire for a child was related to their partner's desire. They wanted a child for "her," because "She would be much happier, and that would in turn make us happier," as one man stated. However, 94% of the women defined their desire to have children and become a family in terms of the continuity of life; creating a family was the real meaning of life. As one participant reported, "That is what life is meant for, to marry and have children. It's been that way since the time of Adam and Eve. It's nothing one can control and decide you can do without."

Twenty-nine percent of the men noted the importance of having a child because there would be someone to take care of them later in life. They were seriously concerned about being left alone in their old age. For these men, infertility was a double blow, both in the way it affected their life in the immediate present, as well as a threat to their future security. None of the women mentioned a concern that not having a child might mean that no family member would be available to take care of them in their old age.

For the women, the loss was more directly experienced in the present. Seventy-eight percent felt unfulfilled as women; their psychological and social identity was threatened in daily life. As one woman noted: "When there is a party and all the women start to talk about babies, I just sit there like a big nothing." Sixty-one percent of the women talked about their "natural mother-feelings," and their feelings of loss because they did not have a child with whom to express these feelings. "I have got such strong mother-feelings, and nobody to express them to," one woman said, and she spoke for many of the women. This strong desire to become a mother could well be described as a "passionate attachment to motherhood" (Raphael-Leff, 1992). For these couples, the expected and longed-for child would have been an automatic "open sesame" to the next stage of life. When the child did not arrive, these women were left on the threshold of a closed door; for most an extremely sad and taxing period.

Some ppl want children (& s) but cant.
Sum not possible can hav children but cht want 2.

The Couple and the Social Network

The next stage of life, moving from couple to family, not only includes a change in individual identity, but also has significance for the way in which the couple participates in their social network. Not having a child is defined as not having the 'correct ticket' that allows them full membership of their community. Couples feel alienated from and out of step with their peers (Meyers et al., 1995), "Caught in the 'not-yet-pregnant' state"(Greil, 1991), and burdened with the social disability of infertility (Menning, 1988).

Rosengren (1991), in an ethnology of family-life in the same geographical area from which the sample for this study was drawn, observed that family was the very heart of the community:

> The existence of Asketorp is built around the family–she and he and the children, and everything that has to do with the community of children is more or less everybody's concern. Such events include the last day of the school year, when the whole town is filled with neat children in freshly pressed summer clothes, and the Walpurgis Night celebrations when families gather in some traditional place and celebrate with a

bonfire and fireworks. The celebration of St. Lucia, which has all the characteristics of a beauty contest for the local girls, as they compete for the role of the Saint, and the Christmas Market when the village square is jammed with people and the children are eager to see Father Christmas. For those who have no family it can in the long run be hard to live in Asketorp. (author's translation)

The childless couples in this study confirmed that noted by Rosengren's analysis when they discussed the difficulties of being childless members of the community and its public life, especially family-oriented celebrations and holidays. Participation in such activities was difficult for the childless couple who longed for a child; avoiding these events meant social isolation. Activities that they had happily enjoyed as long as they could remember were gradually becoming more and more painful for them.

One wife who was very much part of the community in which her husband had been born and bred, commented on this by saying:

> All the joy has gone out of these parties and the traditions we've had. We sit by the May-pole like an old couple–smiling stiffly at others' children and eating our cakes.

One man expressed the same thought in the following way:

> It's like there are invisible gates for me. So many things I cannot participate in, having no children. Strange–only two years ago I did not think of it. Silly really, but I would love to be able to go and collect my little boy from football matches, or go to a P.T.A. meeting.

Viewed from a social network perspective, these experiences are ones in which the couples feel a loss because they are unable to make that valued transition from a couple to a family. Well-known social activities have become painful, acting as a mirror for the difference between what they desire in life and the life they are actually experiencing.

Home Ownership

Home ownership was of central importance in the social network to which these couples belonged and 93% of these couples were homeowners. The home represented an important and clearly defined part of their planned evolution from couple to family. Many spoke of how the location and planning of their home was made with children in mind.

Household tasks were a highly valued activity and people took great pleasure in taking care of their homes. Many of the women reported that household activities occupied most of their spare time–and this was told with pleasure. The men were often involved in projects such as adding a room, building a green-house, painting or repairing. Throughout the discussion of the planning, decorating and care of their home was the underlying theme of the desire for children. The spacious rooms, the care and attention that was put into the choice of textiles, furniture, ornaments and gardens, were indicators of life oriented around the home, and family. Some couples had already prepared a room for the baby.

The homes were not only used for rest and relaxation, but were often the center of a great deal of creative activity. Many individuals were employed in work places where the scope for influencing and being creative was limited; spare-time activities compensated for this. Examples of these activities included complicated hand-crafts such as petit-point embroidery (in a few cases practiced even by men), the making of garden-gnomes and trolls, and the crocheting of (matching) bathroom mats, toilet covers and even covers in shapes of poodles or other objects to hide the spare role of toilet paper, not to mention extremely well-tended and beautiful gardens, often with an attendant greenhouse.

Home and the Social Network

Many of the creative activities that centered on the home were also social activities, in that they drew members of the social network together. The couple was often involved in an intricate network of relationships, involving friends and family, often for the purpose of helping each other. Frequently the network gathered around certain household tasks. This could be centered around the butchering, cleaning, packing and freezing of meat from a cow, pig, deer or elk, to be shared by members of the network. Other examples might be cutting down trees to provide for the year's supply of fire-wood, or renting and operating machines such as gardening-tools.

Women also met together to chat and do handicrafts (sewing-circles, for example); they often got together to do activities with their children. The childless couples expressed a feeling of loss during these activities, and the women, in particular, started to experience feelings of being left out or deviant compared to their relatives and peer-group. These feelings were strengthened whenever female members of the network met, as the usual topics for conversation at such gatherings were husbands, children, child-related activities and other general aspects of family-life.

Involuntary Childlessness and the Social Network

Involuntary childlessness can affect most areas of life. However, the effects appear to be more directly felt and are more far-reaching for women than for men. Motherhood seems to be one of the pillars upon which female identity rests, and fertility, the ability to give birth to a child, is the usually taken for granted key to achieving this part of a woman's psychological and social identity (Russo, 1976; Domar, Bromme, Zuttermeister, Seibel & Friedman, 1992; Wirtberg, 1994).

In the rural area with a relatively stable population, from which this sample of couples was drawn, the norm of home and family is very strong. Thus the couples belong to a social context where their (involuntary) childlessness makes them somewhat deviant, both for themselves and others. This was experienced in various ways and in many cases was the source of a great deal of pain.

Couples have to decide whether they will be secretive or open about their infertility to members of their social network. Families and friends start to ask questions when the expected baby fails to arrive (Meyers et al., 1995). If couples choose to be secretive, they take the risk of being exposed to insensitive comments. Nearly all couples described how they had experienced pressure from friends, relations and workmates to have a baby: "What are you waiting for?" and "Isn't it about time, soon?" were two typical kinds of comment. One more hurtful kind of comment was: "Don't you know how to go about it? I can show you!", which is one example of a whole range of comments which hinted at the couple's sexual capacity, and in particular that of the men. Other kinds of comment were: "I suppose you are too frugal to have children," or "You should consider yourself lucky that you can have time for yourself."

These comments may have been unintentionally cruel, but they still hurt. However, when choosing to be open about their situation, the couples often found themselves the target of well-intended advice such as, "Adopt and you get a baby in no time," "Relax," "Go away on a holiday and don't think about it" or even, "Get a dog." These comments were particularly hurtful when given by the medical profession when the couple sought help. Then, they felt genuinely misunderstood.

However, as time went on the couples reported that such comments, whether intentionally cruel or not, dried up, and that people in their network instead seemed to become rather careful about talking about babies in their presence. If the comments had hurt, so did the silence, and the couples, and in particular, the women, felt an increasing isolation. It was as if they became "disconnected" from their network in some fundamental way.

Non-Mothers and Non-Fathers

One of the differences between women and men in respect to their involuntary childlessness was that for the women there were no "pain-free" zones. Everything and everyone served to remind the women of their undesired state; the experiences for men, however, tended to be compartmental-ized. Although men were aware of their childlessness at home, particularly in the presence of their wife, work was a relatively peaceful place, where they could think about quite different things, together with their friends and col-leagues.

The initial experience of being childless was rather different for men than for women. Even though they wanted a family, men did not initially experi-ence the loss in personal terms. Rather, they experienced the loss as a re-sponse to their wife's experience. For the men the phenomena of childless-ness was very much linked to their partners and the ways in which the partners responded. Thus, the women had specific reactions towards their childlessness; the men, in turn, reacted to their partners' reactions–a some-what simplified view, but one that accurately reflected the general pattern described by the couples in the interviews.

Infertility and childlessness became most painful in the presence of other women; relationships with their sisters, mothers and friends became strained because of their childlessness. They felt more and more excluded from their family of origin, and believed that they were valued less and less. In some cases the pressure was overt. Parents expected their adult children to have babies to continue the family line. In other instances, the pressure was covert; siblings who produced children became more attractive to parents than their childless brothers and sisters.

Several women complained that since they had no children they were always the ones who were expected to be accommodating regarding the time and place for family gatherings. "We are the ones who are expected to travel and fit in our lives to theirs as soon as we shall meet because we don't have children," one woman complained.

The childless women were also expected to help out more with their parents, as they "had no children to worry about." Burns (1987:358) notes that the boundaries between family members seem to become less clear when adult children fail to produce a family of their own:

> Changing loyalties are a part of adulthood that often becomes confused and muddled for the infertile couple. When they are childless, a hus-band or wife may remain torn in their loyalties between their families of origin and their spouses, thus becoming a marginal person in their marriage.

Women and Friends

An obvious sore spot with the women, one which they wanted to spend a lot of time discussing with the interviewer, was change that had occurred in the relationships with female friends. Forty-seven percent of the women stated that they wanted to be able to discuss the changes that have occurred because they were infertile with their female friends. These women had long-term friendships with girlfriends whom they had followed through the different phases of life. However, their friends now had children or were pregnant, and this highlighted the childless women's situation. Friendships became strained and many women reported that these long-time friends avoided them. They felt left out and in some cases, other women replaced them as friends. "I am no good any more," one woman reported, "because she cannot natter with me for hours about feeding bottles and nappy-rashes." Ambivalence and anger as a result of changes in the status of friendship was reported by 50% of the women. These women felt socially handicapped by their unwanted childlessness and excluded from the course of life.

Women at Work

In the study, all but one of the women were in paid employment and 29 of the 30 women were employed in places where their colleagues were predominantly female such as hospitals or day-nurseries for children. This work has little social status and few opportunities for professional development. Therefore, one way of making oneself special was to talk about one's private life.

The principal topic for discussion among women at work was children, or child-related issues. "Children-stories" were the most favorite topic during work-breaks, and as a result colleagues got to know each other's children well, and became involved with them, even though they might never have met them.

For the involuntarily childless woman it was easy to feel (and even be) excluded from this "society of mothers." One woman summed up this situation, saying, "I feel awful when the women at work say that people with no children should have no opinions on child-rearing. I feel like I am worth nothing."

Men as Husband-Father

When thinking in terms of gender, it seems that one central and important aspect of male identity in relation to their female partners is to be able to perceive themselves as the provider, in both a material and an emotional sense of the term. In connection to infertility and childlessness it was very clear that the men took, or rather tried to take, a great deal of responsibility for their wives' emotional well-being. In conversations with the men, their role identity as husband was much more dominating than that of their prospective role as father, and the impact of infertility was felt more immediately for them as husbands than as fathers.

The husbands tended to define themselves as less troubled and less affected by being childless than their wives. They were aware of their wives' distress and often tried to support them in various ways. However, such attempts were not always successful, and as a result the men frequently felt at a loss about what they should do. When established (and previously successful) helping strategies such as comforting, trying to be cheerful, "looking on the bright side," or suggesting practical solutions did not have the desired outcome, the men felt helpless. Their failure to relieve their wives of their pain generated feelings of inadequacy. They were unable to provide what any good husband should–an environment in which their partner felt happy and contented. One man said:

> These years have been hell for me, but I try not to show anything. Nothing will be better if I load my problems on to her. I feel such pity for her and when she gets depressed or very emotional about it I try to comfort her and calm her down. I have the ability to be more rational about it and sort out problems. I also try to point out the positive sides but she only gets furious with me although I'm only trying to help her. So as a result of this I get more withdrawn and I escape to my interests and activities.

Many of these men stated that they feel as if they are balancing on a tightrope; if they were to relax for even a moment, they could slip down into chaos and pain. The source of their stress was their wife and her feelings. They wanted to protect her, to do all in their power to shelter her from the cruel world. This meant, of course, that they could not address their own personal thoughts or feelings around being childless. Many of the men explained how they did not dare explore their feelings about children and family with their wives because they did not want to upset them. In this way, the 'childless man' was much harder to get to know than was the 'husband of the childless wife.'

Men and Women Have Different Stories to Tell

The couples were asked a number of specific questions about their experience with infertility and childlessness as well as how they thought that their partner would answer the same question. The questions asked explored the following areas: grief, sorrow, self-pity, anxiety, guilt, anger, self-esteem, sexuality and experiences in relationship to their social network. On all dimensions the men gave significantly more correct answers than their spouses. The men had more accurate knowledge of their partners' feelings and experiences than the women had of their own feelings. Interestingly this did not correlate with the men's own concept of themselves. The men were often hesitant in answering, saying they were not at all sure. This uncertainty, coupled with their reluctance to initiate or even partake in discussions because of the pain it would cause their partner, meant that their knowledge was invisible for their wives, and thereby failed to serve as the support and resource it could have been in the relationship.

On the other hand, the women answered with more assurance concerning how they believed that their partner experienced their situation, claiming that they knew their partner's feelings well, "even though he doesn't really talk about it." These unchecked assumptions–which they 'knew' to be correct–often led to disappointments and misunderstandings.

The ability to talk and share experiences is one obvious way of enriching and developing a relationship, especially when it is necessary to adapt to unwanted circumstances. Differences concerning the men's and women's attitude towards discussing their situation was striking. The women had a definite need to talk about and to share their sadness and grief. Being able to share their sadness served as a source of relief and eased the pain and the difficulties. Unfortunately, for men this created pain. For the women, talking was a meaningful activity and valued as a supportive function in itself. For men, talking about the infertility situation and its related topics had a value only if it could be a means to reach a goal. If the goal was unreachable, discussing this was not only meaningless, but it could have a negative value since it left them unsure of how to console or comfort their wives. "You don't get children by talking," was a comment that many of the men said in the interviews when this topic was discussed.

In failing to talk about such an important issue, the couple can easily burden each other with unchecked assumptions producing feelings of a lack of support and loneliness. One interesting fact that emerged was that when answering the questions about how they perceived each other's experiences, the 'wrong' answers revealed that the men tended to overestimate the degree of their wife's negative experience, while the women tended to undervalue the impact of the negative experience on their partner. This meant that the men believed that their wives suffered more than they actually suffered, while the women tended to think that their husbands were less affected by being childless than they actually were.

Another difference was that the women seemed to suffer because of what they experienced as a threat to their own identity–a threat actualized in the relationships that constitute their social network. Their husbands, on the other hand, were more immediately sensitive to their wife's experience, and suffered with them. Unlike their wives, the men did not experience their social roles of husbands, men, or prospective fathers to be threatened by their participation in the same network. A partial explanation for this is that many of the social activities that men were involved in, such as sports-clubs, helping members of the network with house-building, repairing cars, gardening, etc., were not defined as being directly connected with their role as prospective fathers. This explanation only holds true, however, if we accept that men define themselves and the activities in which they participate differently than women do since all of the above activities can easily be connected to families and family-life, and hence children. As noted above, the men tend to compartmentalize different areas of life, which meant that house-repairs could be thought of as simply house repairs, and did not set in motion thoughts about the children that they did not have (Hansson & Wirtberg, 1995).

For the women, life was experienced differently. Their childlessness spilled into all aspects of life; into their roles as women, wives, daughters, friends, work colleagues and so on. Participation in any social activity was tinged with more or less threat–the threat of being reminded that they had failed to be "normal," and achieve that which could give their lives meaning, and validate them as women. No child means no family; no family results in a real crisis of meaning and identity.

CONCLUSION

Involuntary childlessness affects a fairly large number of couples. Since the effects of involuntary childlessness have major consequences, it is of value to have knowledge of infertility and its psychological and social effects, especially since it appears that men and women experience their situation differently. The experiences that people have when they are unable to develop from a couple to a family because of obstacles beyond their control, has been described.

The couples in this study had a clear definition of what a family was; for them it necessarily included children as a critical part of their relationship. When they were confronted with the possibility that they might not be able to become a family, then their lives were disrupted. Men and women seem to experience this disruption of their lives in very different ways. The women were focused on the nonexistent child and the meaning of the loss of motherhood both on an individual and social level. The concept of 'mother' and the concept of 'woman' became fused together, and grew to have the same meaning. It also affected the women's experience in nearly all contexts (from dreams to social gatherings). Her loss became complex and revealed many facets. Her spouse mainly experienced the problem in terms of how he needed to interact with her.

Once the decision to start a family was made, it was hard to redefine the form of their future life in light of their possible infertility. A complicating aspect of the problem for many couples was the lack of a definitive message from the medical establishment that children were an impossibility; of the thirty-one couples only three knew with certainty that they could never have children together.

This uncertainty is also compounded by the possibilities inherent in a rapidly developing medical technology designed to assist nature. Knowledge of this technology also breeds another uncertainty, as its availability varies not only among, but even inside countries. Frequently, access to new technology depends on the couple's own ability (as well as that of their doctor) to be up-to-date on developments, as well as being able to meet financial demands. Uncertainty, coupled with the strength and urgency of the couple's desire, often created a crisis situation. Couples found themselves in a situation that was difficult to cope with as individuals, as couples, and as members of a social network. The couples here could be likened to "families without children." Not that they filled the traditional view of what a family is, but from an epistemological point of view they were in a kind of name-less state where their daily experiences of life, and what they wanted life to be, were in conflict. From the couple's own point of view they were no longer "just couples" but they were "not yet families" and they had no real control over whether they were ever going to become families in a traditional sense. One woman expressed this dilemma in the following way: "It's like walking into a black hole that has no name and no recognized existence. Once there, there is no way to get back and there is no way to go forward. You can only hope that it will be all right one day."

REFERENCES

Bateson, G. (1980). *Mind and nature: A necessary unity.* Glasgow: Flamingo.

Burns, L. H. (1987). Infertility as a boundary ambiguity: One theoretical perspective. *Family Process, 26*(3), 359.

Carter, E. A., & McGoldrick, M. (Eds.) (1988). *The changing life cycle: A framework for family therapy* (2nd ed.). NY: Gardner Press, Inc.

Dariiluk, J. C. (1988). Infertility and inter-personal impact. *Fertility and Sterility, 49*(6), 982-990.

Domar, A. D., Bromme, A., Zuttermeister, P.C., Seibel, M., & Friedman, R. (1992). The prevalence and predictability of depression in infertile women. *Fertility and Sterility, 58*(6): 1158-1163.

Greil, A. L. (1991). *Not yet pregnant.* New Brunswick, NJ: Rutgers University Press.

Hansson, K., & Wirtberg, I. (1995). Familjen sedd från manligt och kvinnligt perspektiv. (The family seen from a male and female perspective.). *Nordisk Psykologi, 47*(1), 45-60.

Keeney, B. P. (1983). *Aesthetics of change.* NY: The Guilford Press.

Kraft, A. D. P. J., Mitchell, D., Dean, C., Meyer, S., & Wright-Scmidt, A. (1980). The psychological dimensions of infertility. *American Journal of Orthopsychiatry, 50*, 618-628.

Lalos, A. (1985). *Psychological and social aspects of tubal infertility: A longitudinal study of infertile women and their men.* Unpublished doctoral dissertation, Umeå University, Sweden.

Menning, B. E. (1988). *Infertility: A guide for the childless couple* (2nd ed.). NY: Prentice Hall.

Meyers, M., Diamond, R., Kezur, D., Scharf, C., Weinshel, M., & Rait, D. (1995). An infertility primer for family therapists: Medical, social, and psychological dimension. *Family Process 34*(2), 219-231.

Pengelly, P., Inglis, M., & Cudmore, L. (1993). *In search of an imagined future: Infertility and counseling for couples.* Unpublished report, Tavistock Institute for Marital Studies, London.

Raphael-Leff, J. (1992). *Transition to parenthood: Infertility and adoption.* London: Post Adoption Centre.

Rosengren, A. (1991). *Två barn och Eeget hus: Om kvinnor och måns viirldar I småsamället. (Two children and a house of ones own: The worlds of men and women in the small community.)* Unpublished doctoral dissertation, Stockholm University, Carlssons, Stockholm, Sweden.

Russo, N. F. (1976). The motherhood mandate. *Journal of Social Issues, 32,* 143-153.

Trost, J. (1989). Goddag yxskaft! *Fokus på Familjen, 2,* 115-121.

Wirtberg, I. (1992). *His and her childlessness.* Unpublished doctoral dissertation, Karolinska Institutet, Stockholm University, Sweden.

Wirtberg, I. (1994). Den barnlösa familjen. (The Childless Family.) *Fokus på Familjen, 1,* 24-34.

Lithuania:
The Case of Young "Socialist" Families in the Context of Rapid Social Innovation

Alina Zhvinkliene

INTRODUCTION

In both Western and Soviet societies in the 1970s it became obvious that significant changes were taking place in the organization of patterns of family life. Both societies were experiencing a higher frequency of divorce, a shortened length of marriage, increases in single-parent families, and a larger number of single people. Moreover, Western and Soviet societies have experienced decreases in family size and birth-rates, and more liberalized sexual relations, the latter of which has had the important consequence of a dramatic increase in adolescent birth rates and teenage motherhood. Finally, these changes in the organization of family life have been defined in both societies as a family crisis that has promoted moral decay within society.

This specter of family crisis has stimulated numerous sociological investigations within the former USSR. Special attention was focused on younger families, because society's expectations to improve the quality of life in the former USSR were linked to them. In addition, the young family was considered to be most susceptible and sensitive to social environmental effects because its inherent links are in the formative stages.

YOUNG FAMILIES IN LITHUANIA

To test some of these general observations and obtain a description and definition of young families at the moment of social and political change, I

Alina Zhvinkliene can be reached at Seskines 63-5, 2010, Vilnius, Lithuania.

[Haworth co-indexing entry note]: "Lithuania: The Case of Young 'Socialist' Families in the Context of Rapid Social Innovation." Zhvinkliene, Alina. Co-published simultaneously in *Marriage & Family Review* (The Haworth Press, Inc.) Vol. 28, No. 3/4, 1999, pp. 135-144; and: *Concepts and Definitions of Family for the 21st Century* (ed: Barbara H. Settles et al.) The Haworth Press, Inc., 1999, pp. 135-144. Single or multiple copies of this article are available for a fee from The Haworth Document Delivery Service [1-800-342-9678, 9:00 a.m. - 5:00 p.m. (EST). E-mail address: getinfo@haworthpressinc.com].

135

conducted a longitudinal sociological investigation in the city of Vilnius, Lithuania between 1984 and 1985. The sample was drawn from young couples who submitted their applications for marriage registration and agreed to participate in the research. The marriage applicants, who were of Lithuanian cultural background, under the age of 30, and not previously married, were contacted. The study consisted of two stages, with 220 couples being questioned before marriage and 200 couples after the first year of marriage. Of the 200 married couples, about 90% had participated in the study prior to marriage.

Some Characteristics of the Newly-Weds

The marriage applicant data set provides a picture of the characteristics and activities of young couples. A third of the young married became acquainted during such leisure activities as discotheques, cafes, hikes, etc. A quarter knew each other from childhood or lived in the same house or street, 3% had become acquainted through their parents, 7% by meeting at work, and 20% by studying together. The length of courtship before deciding to marry varied from about 8% who married after knowing each other for less than a month to 20% who had dated for over three years. The length of courtship for the remainder of the sample fell between these two extremes with 27% having dated for 3-6 months, 22% dating for about a year, and 23% dating for more than a year before marriage.

The frequency of dates before deciding to marry was fairly intense with about 37% meeting almost daily and 30% several times a week. Only a third of all the respondents limited their dates to several times per month. Such frequent contact is not surprising, because their mutual interest would make one strive to meet the chosen one more frequently.

Especially young men (33%), but also young women (21%) reported that attractiveness was the most important criterion for choosing a partner. Young men's responses tended to reflect such characteristics as "very beautiful," while girls tended to list characteristics such as "attractive," or "my ideal." The second important criterion for 24% of men and 22% of women was having similar personality needs, common interests and tastes. Finally, a fifth of the men and a fourth of the women could not identify specific characteristics and reported their reasons as "liked," "fell in love," "don't know," etc.

Another focus was a comparison of the individuals' motives for marriage and how this affected their courting behavior before marriage. It was believed that motives for marriage and related courtship behavior might provide important insights into future marital stability. Seventy percent of the men and 63% of the women gave as the main reasons for wanting to marry "a wish to love and be loved," "a wish to have children," or "a wish to have their own house." These motives for marriage are critical for newly-weds, because society places a high value, in regards to marriage, on these norms and values. These motives increased in importance during the first year of marriage with 82% of all young spouses providing such reasons for deciding to have a family.

Motives such as "fear of loneliness," and attitudes indicating a belief that "single people are less valued in the society," reflect the social prestige of marriage in our thinking and behavior. The percentage of women identifying these motives is almost half as much again as those of men, a finding that may reflect traditional negative attitudes towards non-married women as "old maids."

A fifth of the respondents noted that the pregnancy of the bride stimulated family creation and marriage. This reason was linked, however, to negative premarital expectations for the happiness of the would-be family. Almost half the respondents had no faith in the future successfulness of the family when pregnancy was a motive for marriage.

Although young people are often guided by emotional criteria when being motivated to choose a spouse, only about half of the newlyweds (60% of men and 49% of women) are sure that their marriage will be happy. Only 5% of all respondents hope for success and some 10% of men and 20% of women do not think their needs will be satisfied in their marriage. For quite a number of young people, the creation of their first family may be a tribute to the high social status of marriage, not to their own estimates of success.

Characteristics of Young Families After Marriage

The data reflecting the ideas of young spouses concerning the situation in their families suggest that young Lithuanian families may be characterized as follows:

- A low level of cultural communication is observed that manifests itself in low tolerance within the sphere of personal contact on the part of both spouses. Only a quarter of all respondents report that they have never argued. The rest report that they frequently engage in conflict because of excessive drinking or tobacco use, as well as housekeeping conflicts.
- Reciprocity in the egalitarianism of spouses is observed concerning the question of leadership in the family. The majority of respondents suggested that various family life problems were considered together, but decisions often considered the opinion of the particular spouse who was thought to be most competent in a given area or situation. For Lithuanian families, a tradition of equal rights is maintained, but it appeared that housekeeping responsibilities followed a traditional division of home-household obligations for a third of the couples who were ques-

tioned. The rest said they kept house together–an opinion reported equally by men and women.

- Leisure time activities are mostly devoted to family activities outside the home. Sixty percent of all the respondents answered that they like to spend their leisure time in public places, attending various cultural events, while a fifth of young husbands and a quarter of young wives prefer staying-at-home.
- A young family, as a rule, is still economically dependent and does not have its own household. Only a tenth part of the respondents noted having separate floor-space. Most young families at the beginning of the second year of their marriage live with their parents. Half of all the respondents live with the wife's parents and problems in the relationship between the spouses are often thought to occur because of the wife's parents rather than because of the husband himself. Moreover, young couples often make use of material help from their parents, with continued material help being received by a third of the respondents. Almost half of all the respondents are given such help in the case of need.
- Grandparents as an important source of help with household management were identified by 30% of wives and 21% of husbands. Grandparents also assist in childrearing, with 15% of the respondents noting that their parents provide considerable help for a young family. Another 15% percent of the respondents reproached their parents for not helping them with their children, although 25% noted that at times they are looking for such help. Most newly-wed parents, however, often reject moral help from parents, with 60% reporting that they do not need their parents' advice.

The Image of a Successful Marriage

The second goal of our research was to examine factors represented by the images that are connected with various aspects of family-marriage relations. These images often have considerable influence on the development of young families.

We have divided the images of marriage into "normative, generally accepted stereotypes," and "individual, pragmatic, expectations." The latter, as a rule, occurs prior to marriage and forms personality expectations related to marriage. These expectations reflect the way the partners see marriage as the mechanism for realizing one's psychological, physiological, social, and other needs during marriage. These expectations depend somewhat on the stereotype that corresponds to them. Such stereotypes contain directions for the performance of standardized, regulated roles and family functions for both spouses. These premarital expectations are influenced by the existence of the potential spouse and are integrated into the expectations for successful family

life from the other spouse's perspective. Correspondingly, the level of realization of premarital expectations affects the development of young marriages and becomes integrated into marital assessment. Moreover, the character of developing marriage and family relations in a young family depends,
not so much on the expectations of each spouse that are linked with family
realization, but rather on the compatibility of the partner's expectations.
Positive evaluations of both spouses' expectations as relates to marriage are
perhaps a guarantee of stability in marriage.

Cramer's coefficient was used in estimating the interrelated properties;
compatible properties at the 95% level of significance was V = 0.13. In
future-marriages, the expectation that heads of a family will use an egalitarian distribution of authority is related to the expectation of successful family
life (V = 0.18). As a result of gaining family life experience at the beginning
of the second year of marriage, the rather abstract notion (under contemporary social conditions) of "the head of one's family" has begun to be given
concrete expression through the spouses' everyday interaction.

The successful realization of family life expectations and estimation of
marriage depends on:

1. Whether or not the budget distribution in the family is egalitarian (V =
   0.37);
2. How disagreements are resolved, with more than half of the respondents yielding to each other during disagreements (V = 0.27);
3. The degree of satisfaction with the choice of a spouse, with one-fourth
   of the respondents thinking that if they had another choice they would
   reject the present spouse (V = 0.26);
4. Material help to the married couple from the wife's parents, with most
   respondents being given such help (V = 0.26);
5. The character of intimate life, with almost half of the respondents noting problems in this area (V = 0.22);
6. The date of child-birth, with 43 percent of all the young families questioned having already had children by the beginning of the second year
   (V = 0.18).

Such seemingly significant factors, however, like budget size and the size
dwelling places appear to have no effect on the evaluation of marriage of
young families. A possible reason for such results is that changes in the
material-everyday life conditions of young families appear to be expected.

If successful family development is to be better understood according to
sequences of manifestation, the absence of interrelationships between premarital expectations and various aspects of family-marriage relations and
those of successful family life must be examined. Of particular note is the
expectation that the head of the family has little impact on the expectation of

successful family life, whereas the estimation of the marriage by both spouses greatly depends on whether their opinions are reciprocal. The creation of the marriage may be stimulated by social motives and then preserved by the emotional motives.

Social motives dominate the rationales for the creation and structuring of families. Such is the case for first marriage as shown through the structure and sequencing of human life: education, acquisition of a profession, marriage, birth of a child, etc. Undoubtedly, some events may fall out this succession for some families, but, for many, such a pattern of life sequencing is characteristic of former and, probably, future young generations.

A CHILD AT THE BEGINNING OF THE MARRIAGE

The birth of a child or several children is seen as the necessary attribute of family life within common social norms. Consequently, not one of the spouses in this research declared a preference for being childless. At the same time, about one-fifth of all premarital respondents indicated that the bride's pregnancy was a motive for family creation, while more than a quarter of the respondents were expecting a child during their first year of marriage.

Despite this motive for family formation, an interrelationship between reproductive expectations and successful family life expectations does not exist in a practical sense. One exception is help from their own parents in attending and bringing up children–help which is expected to be temporary. A relationship that is almost significant ($V = 0.14$), however, suggests that for some young families, the birth of a first child at the beginning of marriage seems to limit their expectations for a successful family life. Consequently, success is defined, to some degree, by the extent to which the young parents have some freedom from tending to a newborn. That is, the timing rather than the fact of child-birth seems to have an effect on the evaluation of marriage.

The presence of a child in the family seems to affect the following variables:

1. The person who initiates leisure most often is the husband ($V = 0.15$);
2. The character of the division of everyday duties is more often egalitarian and is related to receiving help from parents ($V = 0.14$);
3. Attitude towards budget distribution more often reflects a lack of material resources ($V = 0.15$);
4. Attitudes towards material help often reflect the need for more permanent material help ($V = 0.15$);
5. Young families more often note problems in the intimate aspects of family life ($V = 0.13$).

Although differences in family images may exist between families with and without children, little evidence suggests that children influence the compatibility between spouses. This lack of a role for children in the images of young spouses is confirmed indirectly by their answers to an open-ended question concerning the reasons that influence the success of families or their disintegration. Commonly, children take a fourth place in the hierarchy of primary reasons for family preservation, whereas childlessness as a reason for breaking up a family takes only 7th-8th place in this hierarchy. This relationship is the same both prior to and following marriage.

Although the influence of a child, per se, may not influence compatibility between couples beginning their married life, a child may be a factor affecting the stability or break-up of the marriage. If emotional motives are prevalent in preserving the marriage, the affection felt for a child (or children) may play a role in the marriage. One may theorize, for example, that prior to the development of parental feelings in young parents, they might be more susceptible to marital break-up. The presence of children, in turn, may stimulate the formation of a more monolithic unit and contribute to stability, a finding that is confirmed by recent statistics on divorce within young families.

STEREOTYPES OF FAMILY-MARRIAGE RELATIONSHIPS

Human behavior, especially during critical life situations that require decision-making (e.g., the beginning of intimate life, a decision to have a family, give birth to children, to divorce, etc.), is guided by normative or generally accepted images or stereotypes. The most important reason for being guided by these expectations is to avoid or lessen the consequences of conflicts with the direct social environment. Most young people who are going to get married have certain stereotypes about a good husband or wife, the totality of which is being formed during the process of personality socialization.

To study their opinions, couples were asked to name the most important features of a good husband and wife, which, to their opinion, determined successful family life. The answers were grouped as follows: (1) the ability to act; (2) the ability to feel; (3) the stability of feelings; (4) the orientation towards family; (5) intellect; and (6) sexual accordance or compatibility.

The data suggest that younger spouses generally paid more attention to the ideal features noted above when they were newlyweds. However, both younger spouses, and newlyweds in general, believed that it was important that their spouse, but not necessarily themselves, had characteristics demonstrating "the ability to act," "the ability to feel," "the stability of feelings," and "an orientation towards family." "Intellect" and "sexual accordance" were of lesser importance. It appears that respondents demanded that their spouse fulfill these ideals but consider their own personality to be above reproach.

The elements of "double" morality in marriage and family relations have been retained in the premarital images of young Lithuanians; men are allowed liberties that women are not permitted. Although the majority of couples were fairly tolerant regarding premarital sexual intercourse, males having premarital experience was condemned by a fifth of the marriage applicants, while females having premarital experience was condemned by more than a quarter of marriage applicants. Some of the respondents approved of sexual intercourse if it was limited to couples preparing to marry–an important consideration since one-third of the respondents favored banning abortions.

Although it is maintained that experience in intimate life prior to marriage stimulates the infidelity of spouses, a majority of the respondents are expecting absolute fidelity from spouses in marriage. At the same time, adultery is viewed as a form of intimate relations that may accompany marriage. In answers concerning the reasons for divorce, all the respondents assigned first place to infidelity by their spouses, while only a small number of respondents are in favor of restricting divorce. More than a quarter of the respondents accept divorce only if children are not involved, whereas more than a third accept marital dissolution when children are present. Most respondents understand that divorce is a highly conflicted alternative to married life.

Meanwhile, current stereotypes reflect not only the tolerant views in the field of family and marriage, but also the peculiarities of social-economic conditions that modern families must face. More than half of the respondents believe that the mutual orientation of spouses towards family life is an important aspect of a successful marriage. A quarter of the husbands and wives indicate that three conditions are equally important for successful family life: (1) the mutual orientation of spouses towards the family; (2) social assistance from the larger society; and (3) support from parents and relatives, especially in families who have children.

CONCLUSION

This research on 'normal' young families was the first of its type and still the only current one in Lithuania. Current research is mostly directed toward the studies of public opinion in regard to family life in general.

The research data affirmed that one's need for a family and having child(ren) in the family is to a certain extent a personal decision. It shows that the value of marriage is still very great and that family life is often taken into account in evaluating personal needs. Such a conclusion corresponded with the ideology of socialist families. That is, the Marxist-Leninist tradition of the "socialist family" was contrasted with the "bourgeois family" by assuming that heterosexual monogamy should exist based on the "true sex love" between husbands and wives who were "equal." Consequently, by the middle of 1980s, Lithuanian youth had adopted the norms of the "ideal socialist family."

Currently, these norms are not being reinforced in either the official ideology of Soviet society or in Lithuania. The goals of national rebirth were developed as an outgrowth of restoring the traditional gender-structured family of Lithuania, which lost its shape during the Soviet period of Lithuanian history. By the end of 1980s and beginning of 1990s, a sharp critique of Soviet reality provided impetus for people to move towards the liberalization of political and economic life, as well as traditionalism in family life. The New Right's social philosophy (Green, 1986; Diamond, 1995) encourages traditional gender structured families under free market economic policies, a pattern that is similar to the family ideals being promoted in the former USSR. The ideas of the new-familialist (Struening, 1996) of the 1990s correspond more to the Soviet family ideology of the 1970s than do the ideas of the New Right. The new familialist thought is tolerant of "non-traditional" families, but actively promotes heterosexual two-parent families, while supporting equal rights and opportunities for women.

According to public opinion surveys, Lithuanian people are traditionalists in regard to the organization of family life and women's roles. The surname of Lithuanian women, for example, indicates their marital status, which means that women who marry prefer to take their husbands' names, and quite often keep it after divorce.

The number of marriages in Lithuania was relatively stable over the entire Soviet period, but the number of divorces tended to increase and then stabilized during the 1980s. In the period from 1985-90, there were 9.6 marriages and 3.3 divorces per one thousand in the population, whereas by 1994 the number of marriages and divorces dropped to 6.3 and to 3.0 per one thousand in the population (Demographic yearbook: 1994, 1995).

Consistent neo-conservative ideologies, new emphases on national rebirth and the traditional family patterns of Lithuania ideologies (and less emphasis on the Soviet family) have influenced the number of teen marriages and live-births by adolescent mothers. The rate of brides per 1000 females under the age of 20 increased from 44.5 in 1980 to 65.9 in 1990, and decreased again to 47.7 in 1994. The rate of bridegrooms per 1000 males under the age of 20 increased from 14.4 in 1980 to 19.2 in 1990, and decreased again to 15.3 in 1994. The rate of live births per 1000 females aged 15-19 increased from 28.0 in 1980 to 41.6 in 1990 (47.9 in 1991), and decreased again to 41.0 in 1994 (Demographic statistics in the Baltic countries, 1996).

Although the socialist period provided some privileges for single mothers, the number of unmarried live-births was not comparatively high and almost corresponded to the period prior to the Second World War. The ratio of illegitimate children had been between 6% to 7% since the period from 1922 to 1939 and 5% to 7% during the 1980s. In 1994, illegitimate live-births were 10.8% of all live-births in Lithuania and the number of unmarried teen mothers increased by 59% between 1989 and 1994.

A sharp decrease in the total number of marriages and live-births in Lithuania could be one sign that the Soviet period provided a more favorable climate for marriage and having children. Despite the traditional conservatism of Lithuanians during a time of social control and the relatively stable socio-economic circumstances of the Soviet years, family formation with children was more prevalent during the Soviet period than during our present period of liberalization.

Statistical comparisons concerning family liberalization in Lithuania and western countries suggests that there is a "time delay" in family trends that have occurred in western countries reaching Lithuania. The western 'sexual revolution' of the 1960s appears to have reached Lithuania thirty or more years later (Zhvinkliene, 1992). However, as the liberalization of larger political and socio-economic forces continues to liberalize the family institution, the "time delay" between Lithuania and western countries appears to grow shorter (Zhvinkliene, 1997). Consequently, liberal political and social changes in Lithuanian society appear to be making a profound impact, initially, on marital behavior among Lithuanian youth. As a result, greater variety is appearing in the organization of family life, which as yet, has 'escaped' the sociologist's notice in Lithuania.

REFERENCES

Demographic statistics in the Baltic countries (1996). Lithuanian Department of Statistics, Statistical Office of Estonia, Central Statistical Bureau of Latvia, Tallinn, Riga, Vilnius.

Demographic yearbook 1994 (1995). Lithuanian Department of Statistics, Vilnius.

Diamond S. (1995). *Roads to dominion. Right-wing movements and political power in the United States*. New York: The Guilford Press.

Green, D. G. (1986). *The new right: The counter-revolution in political, economic and social thought*. Brighton: Wheatsheaf Books.

Struening K. (1996). Feminist challenges to the new familialism: lifestyle experimentation and the freedom of intimate association. *Hypatia, 11* (1), 135-153.

Zhvinkliene, A. (1992, February). The main features of reproductive behavior in Norway and Lithuania. Report on scholarship presented for the Norwegian Research Council for Science and the Humanities (NAVF).

Zhvinkliene, A. (1997). Family discourse: The case of Lithuania and Finland. In M. Taljunaite (Ed.), *Everyday life in the Baltic States* (pp. 160-171). Institute of Philosophy and Sociology, Republic of Lithuania; University of Goteborg, Center for Russian and East Studies, Sweden.

SECTION III:
FAMILIES AND SUPPORT SYSTEMS

Defining Families
Through Caregiving Patterns

Joan Aldous

INTRODUCTION

In the United States, especially during this last few decades of the 20th century, there are enough types of close living relationships in large enough numbers so that we can literally speak of our subject matter as being the study of families rather than the study of the family. Along with families based on intact marriages with no background of divorce, there are also single-parent families, cohabiting couples, married couples in which one or both spouses have been previously married, and step-families that result from remarriages where children from previous unions are present. With such a variety of groups, most of whose members would insist they are families, it is difficult to give a definition that holds for all. One that I have increasingly used is that *families* are cohabiting groups of some duration, the members of which are

Joan Aldous is affiliated with the Department of Sociology, University of Notre Dame, Notre Dame, IN 46556.

[Haworth co-indexing entry note]: "Defining Families Through Caregiving Patterns." Aldous, Joan. Co-published simultaneously in *Marriage & Family Review* (The Haworth Press, Inc.) Vol. 28, No. 3/4, 1999, pp. 145-159; and: *Concepts and Definitions of Family for the 21st Century* (ed: Barbara H. Settles et al.) The Haworth Press, Inc., 1999, pp. 145-159. Single or multiple copies of this article are available for a fee from The Haworth Document Delivery Service [1-800-342-9678, 9:00 a.m. - 5:00 p.m. (EST). E-mail address: getinfo@haworthpressinc.com].

usually economically dependent on each other. Moreover, they are composed of persons in intimate relations that are based on biology, law, custom or choice (Aldous & Dumon, 1990).

A functional definition of the family circle also may be provided by the helping patterns among individuals, which often take the form of giving and receiving financial aid as well as caring for physical needs. Watching out for each other is one of the intimate aspects linking members into what we identify as a family.

The particular focus of this paper, therefore, is on families' and members' caregiving activities throughout their lives. My concern is with the fairly expectable problems that families face at particular stages of their existence as part of a family development approach (Aldous, 1996). To the extent possible, I shall attempt to provide a sketch of the caregiving challenges that families face over their particular histories. A consideration of family lives will give us an idea of how these capacities vary over time for members of all ages. This schema also includes a discussion concerned with when family members are especially likely to need someone to look out for them. It includes a description of how, over time, families broaden or shrink the boundaries of those they view as members in terms of caregiving. I will conclude with a summary of demographic and social changes that affect caregiving and the persons for whom care is provided.

Definitions

Let me begin by putting family caregiving in perspective and defining some terms. The usual term used for family activities on behalf of ailing or dependent members is caregiving. *Caregiving* refers to the physical work involved but also includes the accompanying comfort that family members provide each other. We count on caring and the carework to which it gives rise as being found in devoted family relations, especially those for which women are responsible (Graham, 1983).

Caring and caregiving are often seen as the defining characteristics of women. Watching over others involves the warm feelings and private activities that persons stereotypically expect women to display in their customary domestic settings (Osmond & Thorne, 1993). In contrast to this traditional depiction of women, men's identity has been seen more often as wrapped up in doing things for themselves and by themselves often in public places (Graham, 1983; Brines, 1994). Men often appear to expect someone to watch over them, and that someone, in most cases, is a woman, usually an intimate other, such as a wife or a daughter. A majority of women, including those with young children who join men in the competitive labor force, are still assigned homemaking responsibilities (Hochschild, 1989). With the responsibilities of caring for children and participating in the paid labor force, who will provide the care that women typically provided? As this paper will document, it is spouses and other women, mothers, sisters or daughters, who care for them. Thus, our interest in family caregiving over time more often has less to do with families than it does with women in families.

It is well to note that, just as the neutral term "caregiving" hides its ties to one gender, our knowledge of when families provide such services obscures reality. In one review of the research on care providers, the authors concluded that "most" of the work on the caregiving burden has concerned "primarily" those who help the frail elderly or dementia patients (Raveis, Siegel & Sudet, 1988-1989). There are good reasons why special attention is devoted to the elderly, one of which being that they are more likely to be infirm. One wonders, however, if the disproportionate numbers of articles and books devoted to their condition may not overlook other members in need of special family caregiving attention.

Before addressing specifics, however, it is important to note that the terms generation and cohort appear in the following analysis. By generation and cohort, I will be referring to the consequences of family time. *Generations* measure time in terms of forebears and descendants–our parents and grand-parents, our children and grandchildren. *Cohort*, in contrast, refers to persons born around the same period within the various families.

FAMILY TIME PERIODS AND THEIR CAREGIVING CHALLENGES

For the purpose of giving an overview of the divisions in family time and their expected caregiving demand, one can demarcate a beginning period when families (of procreation) become started, followed by child bearing and child rearing periods. Children become mature and start leaving home, so that a parent or parents are eventually alone in their middle years to sustain the family. A family of procreation's life ends, in turn, with the aging and deaths of parents marking the final period (Aldous, 1996).

Having delineated divisions in family time, let me now describe these periods in terms of their problematic aspects. In beginning this consideration of stages in family lives and how family caregiving might fit within them, it is well to note that families in the traditional sense, of those being formed through marriage, continue to exist. Despite the rise in cohabitation rates, half of recent marital partners have cohabited, and most persons eventually marry. Among white women born in the 1950s, estimates are that 91 percent will eventually marry, though ethnic differences exist, with the comparable figure for black women being 75 percent (Cherlin, 1992).

If most people do marry, simply staying together is the overriding problem that newlyweds in the beginning stage of family life must address. Well over half (56%) of all persons born in the early part of the 1950s will divorce, a generalization that applies to the vanguard of the baby boomer generation (Norton & Moorman, 1987). Marital break ups occur fairly early in marriage, with 40 percent of the separations taking place less than five years after the wedding day (Bumpass, Sweet & Castro-Martin, 1990).

The difficulty these divorces create for the former partners and their relatives can be considerable. The emotional and economic stress that couples and their kin experience when they split up is accentuated when children are present. In the first half of the 1980s, almost three-fourths (69 percent) of marital separations involved children (Bumpass, Sweet & Castro-Martin, 1990).

Because women's economic status after divorce tends to fall by about a third (30%), remarrying is one means to repair their families' financial situation (Hoffman & Duncan, 1988). Somewhat more than 70% of separated women will remarry after divorce. However, women over 30 and women with children are less likely to remarry (Bumpass, Sweet & Castro-Martin, 1990). These remarriages, in turn, are more likely to dissolve than are first marriages. Among white women married between 1980 and 1985, for example, remarried women were 25 percent more likely to divorce (Castro-Martin & Bumpass, 1989).

We should also not overlook the considerable number of unmarried women in the U.S. who start their families by bearing children. In 1990, 35% of children under 18 who were living in single parent families were living with a never-married parent compared to 37% who were living with a divorced parent (Saluter, 1994). Again, there are racial differences in the likelihood of giving birth as an unmarried parent. In 1993, 20.6% of white women were never-married mothers compared to 2.8% in 1970. In 1993, 55.4% of black mothers had never married as compared to 15.1% in 1970. In 1993, 35.4% of Hispanic mothers had never married; data for the earlier year were not available (Rawlings, 1994).

Poverty more often characterizes these single-mother families, with 39.6% of white single mothers with children under 18 being classified in this manner in 1993. Poverty also characterized 57.7% of black and 60.5% of Hispanic single women householders. (U.S. Bureau of the Census, 1995). This is especially true of unmarried mothers who are less likely to be awarded child support from fathers. For example, in 1992, only 27% of never-married mothers received child support as compared with 66% among ever-married mothers. Moreover, of the custodial mothers who were granted awards in 1991, only a little over half (52.3%) of these women received the full amount and almost a fourth (23.7%) received no payment at all (Scoon-Rogers & Lester, 1995). Thus, single mothers who are responsible for families, whether divorced or never married, are likely to be in financial need. Frequently, if employed, these women face child care problems and, even if well off, they are likely to lack emotional support (McLanahan & Sandefur, 1994).

The middle years often find married couple families in better shape financially to help needy, younger families. However, adult children who either remain at home or return home and stay for a prolonged period of time tend to reduce the amount of time that employed mothers and fathers have to devote to elderly parents (Buck & Scott, 1993; Aquilino & Supple, 1991). If their own marriages are in danger, families in the middle years may be seeking solace from kin who are members of other generations. This is particularly true of women who divorce when their children are reaching adulthood. Although fathers are more apt to lose contact with their children, they are more often sources of comfort to their mothers. Consequently, adult children may also find themselves having to assist mothers who have limited financial resources. This flow of financial resources to middle-aged parents comes from members of the generation that are just beginning to establish their own families and themselves in the employment world. However, in most cases, parents are able to help needy elderly or offspring. There is some evidence that persons who are located between the oldest and youngest living family generations are somewhat more likely to contribute to the former than to the latter. Finally, elderly couples are increasingly characterized by sound enough financial and health circumstances to enjoy their declining years (Aldous, 1995). Frequently, they are able to remain independent and assist their descendants longer before reaching the period of frail health that may make them turn to other family members for care.

To summarize the challenges that families face over the course of their existence, families have a greater challenge with respect to caregiving resources in the formation and child rearing stages. The challenges of maintaining marriages, starting parenthood, divorcing, remarrying and preparing youth to leave home may make these family life stages into 'care seeking' rather than 'care giving' periods. Individuals in the years when children are leaving home are generally better able to handle caregiving demands. Compared to past-times, present-day elderly, except for widows and minorities, are more independent in terms of financial and physical care matters.

MEMBERS' NEED FOR FAMILY CAREGIVING

The family members most in need of help include individuals who are too young or too old to care for themselves. Children are customarily thought of as dependents, because they are presently unable to carry out daily activities without help and supervision. The elderly often fall into this category due to disability; once able to take care of themselves, some may now need help with daily routines. For example, the National Health Interview Survey of

Disability (1983 through 1985) in the United States has defined this circum-stance as being a chronic condition or conditions that prevents individuals from performing the activities of daily living. Such activities include self care, keeping house, working or attending school, depending upon the age of the individual (LaPlante, 1988). This survey also found that somewhat over seven and one-half million persons, or 3.6% of the population, according to this definition, were considered to be disabled.

Age makes a great difference in how many are disabled. Among all per-sons under 25 years of age, less than one percent were in this category (LaPlante, 1988). To keep disability figures according to age in proportion, I should note that the numbers of disabled persons under 65 is substantial (3,207 million), even though the proportion of disabled in the younger group is much less than in the older groups. The total among those 65 and over is 4,369 million or 16.5% of this age group (LaPlante, 1988). The disabled are more likely to have less education, earn lower incomes, and be in poverty than those who are not limited in activities. Those who are 18 years of age and older are also more likely to be in families that are disrupted by death, divorce or separation. As a result, these families are less likely to have members who are able to provide care (LaPlante, 1988).

The Family Caregivers

Having gained some perspective on the persons needing someone to watch over them, let us now turn to the issue "who is actually looking out for them." The touchy area of finances provides an example of the importance of family aid. If we restrict our inquiry only to persons giving regular money payments to individuals living in other households, figures from a national sample demonstrate that very few American families are involved in such financial transfers. Just under four percent (3.7%) of adults in the population who are 18 years of age and over currently give money to about six percent (5.8%) of the population (U.S. Bureau of the Census, 1988). Researchers who have used data from a 1985 national survey, for example, have found that almost 99% of the money going from one household to another has been transferred to relatives (U.S. Bureau of the Census, 1988).

We saw earlier that young families were liable to face the problem of simply staying together along with financial hardships due to higher unem-ployment and lower starting wages. However, it is young adults (25-44) who are most apt to be giving money to another family (i.e., they made up 63% of the givers). These contributors are more likely to be men, with their contribu-tions taking the form primarily of child support payments to the living re-minders of failed marriages. These payments make sense because men earn, on average, more than women and are less likely to have custody of children. Almost half (45.6%) of these men who provide child support were married

(U.S. Bureau of the Census, 1988). Child support, therefore, often appears to flow from one young family to another, with families being defined in terms of parent-child ties.

The same pattern appears with older persons. Individuals ages 45 to 64 who helped other households with money constituted 28% of the givers, with the common patterns being to support parents (50%) more than children (44%) and only rarely both generations. Despite an economic status that is currently better-off, only seven percent of givers were over 65, and in an overwhelming sense, their help went to adult children (U.S. Bureau of the Census, 1988). Men are major supporters of parents as well as children, though daughters and sons give about the same amount to parents (U.S. Bureau of the Census, 1988).

To summarize what we know about the comparatively few financial providers who help other relatives, past marital histories appear to account for the preponderance of younger, presumably less economically advantaged families being involved in such aid. Since these payments take the form of child support, the particularly financially distressed, single-parent families with children are more apt to be recipients of these funds (U.S. Bureau of the Census, 1988).

Aid across family boundaries involves care as well as monetary gifts that enable families to buy care. Information from another recent (1987-1988) national representative sample, for example, provides a useful supplement to what we know about monetary transfers. Interestingly, other forms of aid, such as household services, child care, and emotional support between parents and adult children who live in different homes, showed much the same patterns as financial support. Former members of nuclear families are overwhelmingly involved. Compared to sons, however, daughters are more frequent parties in exchanges with parents, due primarily to their greater receipt of child care and advice. Young parents, who often are economically pressed, are more likely to receive child care and monetary help at this formative stage of the family history (Eggebeen & Hogan, 1990). According to reports from one well-off sample of pre-retirement-aged parents, this is particularly true for the population of divorced women with children who are more likely to be economically disadvantaged. The latter were disproportionately helpful to such daughters who were facing the problematic life of single parents (Aldous, 1985).

Among young families, the most economically deprived group are single mothers with children (especially blacks) who have one or more children under five. Thirty-four percent of young black mothers ages 18-29 live with parents as compared to 21% of young white mothers of similar ages. These young, single-mother families are not receiving substantial amounts of support from their parents, and, contrary to the findings from small scale studies, this is especially true of black mothers. Almost a third of black mothers (31%), and somewhat over a fifth (23%) of white single mothers, receive no parental assistance at all (Eggebeen & Hogan, 1990).

What about intergenerational exchanges with categories of the elderly such as widows and the infirm? The exchange balance in terms of services and money, in this case, does appear to shift toward the benefit of those over 40. Adult children do help more extensively with money and advice when parents are ill; but very old parents and widows who are getting along do not receive much additional financial or other help from children. Moreover, most forms of intergenerational support tend to be episodic and to be concentrated during the specific period of need. Limited support of this kind results from the lack of finances and competing demands faced by potential caregivers. Parents who have a number of children are less apt to help their parents (Eggebeen & Hogan, 1990). Other data also show that middle-aged children often give more comfort and care to parents during illness than they receive themselves. Their elderly parents often reciprocate, in turn, with disproportionate job advice and monetary help (Rossi, A. S. & Rossi, P. H., 1990). Thus, each generation tries to compensate somewhat for the needs of the other generation, whether or not it involves becoming established in the labor market or dealing with failing health. At the same time, each generation maintains enough distance to fulfill its own priorities.

As was noted above about divorced mothers, previous family connections make a difference in the nature of aid across generations. Child support from a non-resident divorced parent constitutes a large portion of financial assistance coming to custodial parents. However, longitudinal data from the Panel Study of Income Dynamics suggests that, when custodial mothers remarry, "sizable reductions" in the absent fathers' payments occur. Absent fathers also tended to enjoy higher standards of living than their children. They appeared to be able to pay more support than they actually gave, and their payments did not increase as their incomes progressed. Thus, not being in residence functioned to weaken the financial contributions of fathers to their children (Hill, 1992).

These intergenerational deficits of divorced fathers also occur for divorced mothers and remarried parents in reference to the care provided to adult children. For example, the National Survey of Families and Households demonstrated that when compared to offspring of never-divorced parents, children of divorce who were over 18 years of age continued to receive less care from parents (White, 1992). The latter provided less advice, child care, transportation, housework, and financial help. Both mothers and fathers who had experienced these circumstances were less attentive to their adult children. Very little of these lessened relationships was due to diminished resources. Instead, weakened parent-child solidarity, as demonstrated by less contact, greater distance, and lower-quality intergenerational ties seemed to account for these findings (White, 1992).

A. S. Rossi and P. H. Rossi (1990), in their representative sample gathered in Boston, Massachusetts, also found that divorced individuals were less a part of families in terms of helping and support. Specifically, divorced fathers did less for children and divorced mothers were less caring of their parents. As a result, such individuals appear to restrict their attentions to themselves rather than extending care to family members. This may be due, in part, to the personal difficulties involved in marital failure.

Reports from adult children in a longitudinal national sample provide further support for these findings about the effects of divorce (Amato, Rezac & Booth, 1995). For example, those with divorced parents were less likely than adult children from intact families to specify their parents as possible sources of help. Moreover, adult children tended to give single-parent mothers more assistance than they received, but, when mothers remarried, the generational help balance moved in the opposite direction. They were as helpful as first-married mothers to their children, but the latter, due, perhaps, to the unclear boundaries of stepfamilies, were less helpful. They were even less tied to divorced fathers through helping exchanges. Both generations gave less to each other than was true of children and fathers in continuing marriages. Thus, as with residential patterns after marriages terminate, divorced fathers are more apt to be outside the networks of children's helping patterns. When divorce has occurred, caregiving between parents and children can be counted on less than caregiving within intact families whose boundaries have never been breached.

The never married, in turn, often have not been members of partnerships for any length of time and lack offspring who typically would be concerned about their welfare. When their parents are no longer able to help, it appears that siblings are the persons to whom these singles turn for care. The feelings of closeness and the shared memories of growing up together are the common reasons why siblings are likely to respond. However, if siblings are themselves elderly or their spouses and children require attention, these individuals are less likely to be reliable sources of help. As I have shown above, caregiving norms hold for parents, spouses and children, with sibling ties being defined more extensively as matters of choice rather than obligations (Bedford, 1995).

Caregivers of the Infirm Elderly

Before leaving this consideration about the need to care for family members and who provides this service, a more specific focus is needed on the caregivers of the many infirm or disabled who are elderly. National survey data demonstrate that over a third (35.6%) of older people who need help to perform at least one important daily activity tend to depend on a spouse. A roughly comparable number of the caregivers (37.4%) are children of the dependent person who requires care. Sixty-two percent of the daughters and 55.6% of the sons were married and progressing through the years when their own children were leaving home (Stone, Cafferata & Sangl, 1987). Almost three-fourths (72.9%) of the persons caring for the disabled elderly, 65 years of age or older, were either a spouse or a child (Stone, Cafferata & Sangl, 1987). Given this specification of caregiving for the disabled elderly, the apparent definition of the family may be defined in terms of marital or parent-child relations.

Although this is the expected pattern, some of the demographic trends referred to above were complicating the lives of these caregivers. First, a substantial number of children had competing family responsibilities. One-fourth of them still had children under 18 at home, and based on the previous discussion, we would predict that some would be helping adult children. Others had experienced the break-up of their marriages. This was true of almost a third of the daughters (14.2% were widowed and 16.2% were separated or divorced); one-fifth of the sons (19.5%) were divorced (Stone, Cafferata & Sangl, 1987). These problems that caregivers are experiencing tend to diminish their ability to provide assistance. We know from other studies that children of the elderly in disrupted marriages tend to perceive less need and to provide less help to elderly parents, due in major part to job responsibilities (Cicirelli, 1983). Thus, marital disruption weakens ties to the previous generation.

Sons are the caregivers of last resort who tend to play this role only when daughters are not available. Given the smaller families of today, in turn, sons are more likely to have to assume this responsibility. A loop-hole in this tendency, however, is that sons are more likely than daughters to have their spouses fill in for them, so that again women are involved. Daughters also provide more overall services than sons, especially in those cases where personal care is required. Understandably, therefore, sons report less stress than daughters that might result either from assisting their elderly parents or from the competing family responsibilities that may result from these involvements (Horowitz, 1985).

Parents' siblings may be pressed into service to supplement the adult child's care-giving efforts for ailing elders. Parents are living longer but they have fewer children and their daughters are now more likely to be in the paid labor force. Moreover, divorce is more common in the younger generation, which gives rise to a set of circumstances that creates complications in the abilities of family members to help the elderly (Cicirelli, 1992). For these reasons, the elderly may be dependent upon siblings, especially on sisters who can compensate for this caregiving gap. Whether or not this is feasible depends upon the sibling's health, prior relations with the unwell person, physical proximity, and the demands that a sibling's children have placed upon them. Because such assistance is less normative, siblings can view this support as more burdensome than do adult children or partners (Reinhard & Horvitz, 1995). For these reasons, the elderly may be less able to count on siblings to help than either a spouse or child.

Defining Families in Terms of Caregiving

If one defines families only in terms of those who help each other in times of trouble, parent-child ties are of greatest importance. In times of substantial divorce rates, it is the parent-dependent child bond that is most crucial. Older parents still consider their adult children part of their family and frequently provide assistance to them. Adult children who are busy with careers, lack partners, and have young children at home are less likely to reciprocate with care.

Middle-aged, hale and hearty individuals are better off and more likely to be married than in the past. If they choose, they can help children and grandchildren with money and services. They are living longer and as a consequence, are more likely to suffer future disabilities due to extreme old age. Presently, their needs for care when becoming elderly may threaten the work-life and competing family responsibilities of their daughters, and to a lesser extent, their sons.

Demographics are changing and it may be that when this cohort of baby-boom parents are replaced by their offspring who are parents of smaller families (i.e., the baby-bust cohort), then fewer daughters or sons will be available to share in the caregiving burden (Easterlin, Macunovich & Crimmins, 1993). In addition, fewer children will be available who are unaffected by troubled marital histories and the attendant emotional, financial, and child care hardships that make concern for others difficult. Furthermore, the aged also will be more likely to have seen the trajectories of their own families disrupted by divorce and to have shifted through remarriage. Finally, elderly men who experience divorce may be increasingly isolated from supportive networks, due to their loss of contact with offspring (Furstenberg, Peterson, Nord & Zill, 1983; Goldscheider, 1990; Aldous, 1990). Siblings, when able, may be called upon to assist the divorced and the never married as well as caring for elderly married individuals whose spouses or children are unavailable.

If we define families in terms of who gives financial aid or physical care to whom, these primary groups would be limited in membership to predominately family members living together during the child-rearing years. Mothers and to a lesser extent fathers if they are present, provide sustenance to the younger generation. Defined functionally in terms of assistance, the family that a person can usually depend on in times of trouble is the parental family.

So in a world growing increasingly impersonal, family membership is a major source of comfort.

Recent family changes that have disrupted family residential patterns have resulted in stripped-down families. Because of divorce and differential mortality rates by gender, the dependable family members for the caregiving of youngsters and adult children may be limited to a single person, a mother. Fathers who live apart, when they do supply aid, generally do so through financial means. However, mothers, along with their spouses when present, may be choosing which intergenerational ties to honor based on the comparative needs of their offspring. Consequently, they may be preoccupied with another offspring's problems and unable to help. Parents, in turn, are less able to count upon their children for aid and this may explain their tendencies to seek support from their siblings as a supplement to members from the family of procreation. Because of their conflicting responsibilities with employment, other families, and their own parents, adult children or partners cannot guarantee succor, security, and a lasting supply of caring relations.

CONCLUSION

Because of high divorce rates in the U.S., family membership and family responsibilities for adults are becoming matters of choice. Despite growing up in a family of origin and having formed their own family of procreation through marriage, the individuals that one might have expected to provide help in times of trouble may not oblige. Family ties are tenuous and not always honored among adults in terms of providing assistance. This is the case among persons who, as children, were once members of the same nuclear family as well as among those persons who were members of step-families while growing up. Mothers are usually the most likely persons to assist the most needy of the younger generation and fathers are linked through child support payments, at least in a monetary sense, to their children. Along with spouses, older persons include children as family whom they count on for support and caring. A last resort, siblings may be called upon based on close ties from their childhood years. Parents and children who shared a home continue to be primary sources of aid, with mothers and their children constituting the bare bones of functioning families that are defined in terms of caregiving.

REFERENCES

Aldous, J. (1985). Parent-adult child relations as affected by the grandparent status. In V. L. Bengtson & J. F. Robertson (Eds.), *Grandparenthood* (pp. 117-132). Beverly Hills, CA: Sage.

Aldous, J. (1990). Family development and the life course: Two perspectives on family change. *Journal of Marriage and the Family, 52*, 571-583.

Aldous, J. (1995). New views of grandparents in intergenerational context. *Journal of Family Issues, 16*, 104-122.

Aldous, J. (1996). *Family careers: Rethinking the developmental perspective.* Thousand Oaks, CA: Sage.

Aldous, J., & Dumon, W. (1990). Family policy in the 1980s: Controversy and consensus. *Journal of Marriage and the Family, 52*, 1136-1151.

Amato, P. R., Rezac, S. J., & Booth, A. (1995). Helping between parents and young adult offspring: The role of parental marital quality, divorce, and remarriage. *Journal of Marriage and the Family, 57*, 363-374.

Aquilino, W. S., & Supple, K. R. (1991). Parent-child relations and parents' satisfaction with living arrangements when adult children live at home. *Journal of Marriage and the Family, 53*, 13-27.

Bedford, V. H. (1995). Sibling relationships in middle and old age. In R. Bleiszner & V. H. Bedford (Eds.), *Handbook of aging and the family* (pp. 201-222). Westport, CT: Greenwood Press.

Brines, J. (1994). Economic dependency, gender, and the division of labor at home. *American Journal of Sociology, 100*, 652-688.

Buck, N., & Scott, J. (1993). She's leaving home: But why? An analysis of young people leaving the parental home. *Journal of Marriage and the Family, 55*, 863-874.

Bumpass, L., Sweet, J. A., & Castro-Martin, T. (1990). Changing patterns of remarriage. *Journal of Marriage and the Family, 52*, 747-757.

Bumpass, L. & Sweet, J. A. (1989). National estimates of co-habitation. *Demography, 26*, 615-625.

Castro-Martin, T., & Bumpass, L. (1989). Recent trends and differentials in marital disruption. *Demography, 26*, 37-51.

Cherlin, A. J. (1992). *Marriage, divorce, remarriage.* Cambridge, MA: Harvard University Press.

Cicirelli, V. G. (1983). A comparison of helping behavior to elderly parents of adult children with intact and disrupted marriages. *Gerontologist, 23*, 619-625.

Cicirelli, V. G. (1992). Siblings as caregivers in middle and old age. In J. W. Dwyer, & R. T. Coward (Eds.), *Gender, families, and elder care* (pp. 84-101). Newbury Park, CA: Sage.

Easterlin, R. A., Macunovich, D. J., & Crimmins, E. M. (1993). Economic status of the young and old in the working age population, 1964 and 1987. In V. L. Bengtson & W. A. Achenbaum (Eds.), *The changing contract across generations* (pp. 67-85). New York: Aldine De Gruyter.

Eggebeen, D. J., & Hogan, D. P. (1990). Giving between generations in American families. *Human Nature, 1*, 211-232.

Furstenberg, F. F., Jr., Peterson, J. L., Nord, C. W., & Zill, N. (1983). The life course of children of divorce: Marital disruption and parental contact. *American Sociological Review, 48*, 656-688.

Goldscheider, F. K. (1990). The aging of the gender revolution. *Research on Aging, 12*, 531-545.

Graham, H. (1983). Caring: A labour of love. In J. Finch & D. Groves (Eds.), *A labour of love: Women, work and caring* (pp. 13-31). London: Routledge & Kegan Paul.

Hill, M. S. (1992). The role of economic resources and remarriage in financial assistance for children of divorce. *Journal of Family Issues, 13*, 158-178.

Hochschild, A. (1989). *The second shift: Working parents and the revolution at home.* New York: Viking.

Hoffman, S. D., & Duncan, G. J. (1988). What are the economic consequences of divorce? *Demography, 25*, 641-646.

Horowitz, A. (1985). Sons and daughters as caregivers to older parents: Differences in role performance and consequences. *Gerontologist, 25*, 612-617.

LaPlante, M. P. (1988). *Data on disability from the National Health Interview survey, 1983-85. An Information Use Report.* Washington, DC: U.S. National Institute on Disability and Rehabilitation Research.

McLanahan, S. & Sandefur, G. (1994). *Growing up with a single parent: What hurts, what helps.* Cambridge, MA: Harvard University Press.

Norton, A. J., & Moorman, J. E. (1987). Current trends in marriage and divorce among American women. *Journal of Marriage and the Family, 49*, 3-14.

Osmond, M. W., & Thorne, B. (1993). Feminist theories: The social construction of gender in families and society. In P. G. Boss, W. J. Doherty, R. LaRossa, W. R. Schumm & S. K. Steinmetz (Eds.), *Sourcebook of family: Theories and methods* (pp. 591-623). New York: Plenum.

Raveis, V. H., Siegel, K., & Sudet, M. (1988-89). Psychological impact of caregiving on the careprovider: A critical review of extant research. *Journal of Applied Social Sciences, 13* (Fall-Winter), 40-80.

Rawlings, S. W. (1994). Household and family characteristics: March, 1993. *U.S. Bureau of the Census. Current Population Reports, Series P-20, No. 477.* Washington, DC: U.S. Government Printing Office.

Reinhard, S. C., & Horvitz, A. V. (1995). Caregiver burden: Differentiating the content and consequences of family caregiving. *Journal of Marriage and the Family, 57*, 741-750.

Rossi, A. S., & Rossi, P. H. (1990). *Of human bonding: Parent-Child relations across the life course.* New York: Aldine De Gruyter.

Saluter, A. F. (1994). Marital status and living arrangements: March, 1993. *U.S. Bureau of the Census. Current Population Reports, Series P-20, No. 478.* Washington, DC: U.S. Government Printing Office.

Scoon-Rogers, L., & Lester, G. H. (1995). Child support for custodial mothers and fathers: 1991. *U.S. Bureau of the Census. Current Population Reports, Series P-60, No. 187.* Washington, DC: U.S. Government Printing Office.

Stone, R., Cafferata, G. L., & Sangl, J. (1987). *Caregivers of the frail elderly: A national profile.* U.S. Department of Health & Human Services, Public Health Service, National Center for Health Services Research & Health Care Technology Assessment. Washington, DC: U.S. Government Printing Office.

U.S. Bureau of the Census. (1988). Who's helping out? Support networks among American families. *Current Population Reports, Series P-70, No. 13*. Washington, DC: U.S. Government Printing Office.

U.S. Bureau of the Census. (1995). Income, poverty, and valuation of noncash benefits: 1993. *Current Population Reports, Series P-60, No. 188*. Washington, DC: U.S. Government Printing Office.

White, L. (1992). The effect of parental divorce and remarriage on parental support for adult children. *Journal of Family Issues, 13*, 234-250.

In-Laws and the Concept of Family

Helena Znaniecka Lopata

INTRODUCTION

Families have traditionally been formulated through birth, marriage or adoption. Literate societies require legal recognition of family relations that provides the base for rules of descent, inheritance of name and property, and whatever rights and obligations are built into family roles. Other forms of recognition for such roles are present in various religious, ethnic, or subcultural groups.

Societies differ as to the connecting lines that define family relationships beyond the nuclear family. Patriarchal and patrilineal systems may regard the wife/mother's family of orientation as lacking any connection to the children she bears for her husband's kinship line. Thus, a woman's mother never enters the role of mother-in-law to her daughter's husband. The principle behind in-law terminology in bilateral family systems, such as the American and European ones, allegedly makes husbands and wives equal in their relations with each other's families. The latter societies include the concept of in-law in consideration of family composition. *The Oxford Universal Dictionary* (1955, p. 1008) provides it with a Christian religious background:

> -in-law. A phrase appended to names of relationship, as father, mother, son, etc., to indicate that the relationship is not by nature, but in the eye of the Canon Law, with reference to the degree of affinity within which

Helena Znaniecka Lopata is affiliated with the Department of Sociology, Loyola University of Chicago, 6525 N. Sheridan, Chicago, IL 60626.

This article is a revision of a paper presented at the XXVI International Committee on Family Research Seminar of the International Sociological Association on the theme of *What is Family?* Oslo, July 29-August 3, 1991.

[Haworth co-indexing entry note]: "In-Laws and the Concept of Family." Lopata, Helena Znaniecka. Co-published simultaneously in *Marriage & Family Review* (The Haworth Press, Inc.) Vol. 28, No. 3/4, 1999, pp. 161-172; and: *Concepts and Definitions of Family for the 21st Century* (ed: Barbara H. Settles et al.) The Haworth Press, Inc., 1999, pp. 161-172. Single or multiple copies of this article are available for a fee from The Haworth Document Delivery Service [1-800-342-9678, 9:00 a.m. - 5:00 p.m. (EST). E-mail address: getinfo@haworthpressinc.com].

marriage is prohibited. These forms can be traced back to the 14th century. Formerly in-law was also used in the sense of step.

Anthropologists, many of whom have been British, distinguish between two kinds of relatives:

> On the one hand there are blood relatives. On the other there are relatives by marriage, known as 'relations-in-law' and 'step-relations.' In legal parlance these are distinguished as 'consanguineous,' and 'affinal relations.' . . . . 'Affinity' or relationship by marriage is the relation between a person and his or her spouse's relations and blood relations' spouses. (Wolfram, 1987: 12)

This paper will provide support for my definition of family: a family is a group of people entered into family relationships by entering the appropriate social roles.

THE MOTHER-IN-LAW

The most important in-law relationship upon which many rituals and allegedly problem situations are focused the world over is that of mother-in-law and the spouses of her children. In fact, it is her relation with a daughter-in-law that draws most comments, mainly because so many societies are patriarchal, patrilineal and patrilocal, so that a woman does not see her son-in-law as often. Communities in which such contact is unavoidable often develop avoidance rituals. Murdock (1949) found that 57 percent of 250 societies he studied contained mother-in-law-son-in-law avoidance norms and an additional 24% practiced modified avoidance. The great variations in in-law relationships can be illustrated with two extreme examples, that of highly patriarchal, patrilineal and patrilocal societies and that of modern America with a very loose set of in-law roles.

The family system that requires a bride to leave her family of orientation and to become totally dependent upon her in-laws is evident in most traditional Oriental cultures. Two frequently discussed examples of extremes of in-law control over a wife are traditional China and in some areas of India of even modern times.

> China's traditional marriage practices included child betrothal, polygyny, and concubinage. Marriage was considered a business arrangement whereby a husband and his mother acquired a virtual 'slave.' . . . A wife was the property of a clan, a bearer of sons, a daughter-in-law. . . . She was there to serve all members of an extended family. When her

husband died, her loyalty and servitude to his family and to her widowed mother-in-law remained. (Barnes, 1987, p. 197)

A frequent, or at least more frequently publicized, recent problem accompanying marriage for women in segments of Indian society is that of "kitchen
fires." Young wives are found burned to death in the home of the husband
and/or his family. The women's organizations and mass media blame the
dowry system for these deaths. Either the wife's family of orientation had not
completed its payment of the agreed-upon dowry, or the in-laws demand
more goods, which the family refuses to pay. Once the wife is dead, the son
can remarry and the family thus gains another dowry. One story that ran in
the Indian newspapers the winter of 1987-8 claimed that the cause of a
specific "kitchen fire" had been a motorcycle that the wife's family refused
to provide. Editorials claimed that such demands were a result of "Western-
ization" or the absorption of material values absent in the past. Not only the
husband but also the in-laws are now being held accountable, and in some
cases punished for such deaths (Khan & Rav, 1984).

Mistreatment by in-laws and related problems were listed as some of the
reasons for prostitution in Delhi, India, according to Pillai (1982: 313). Specifically, these included

> poverty, ignorance, craze for a glamorous life, marriage arranged
> against the girl's wish, negligence or desertion by the husband, ill
> treatment by in-laws, lack of education at school and at home, cruel or
> rude treatment by husband and other relatives, unhealthy environment
> and imitation of Western ways of life.

Further proof of in-law problems among many groups in this heavily
patriarchal society of India are contained in suicide and mental health figures.
Bhatia and associates (1987) found different factors contributing to suicide in
India and the United States. Only in India are disputes with spouse and
in-laws included. Parasuraman (1986) concluded that a major factor leading
to mental illness among young wives in India is being left behind with
in-laws when the husband migrates from rural to urban areas or to other
societies.

One consequence of the power of in-laws in India over the life of a
woman, with an unusual and much publicized twist, is associated with widowhood. Since the bride usually moved in with her husband's family for
religious and cultural reasons, the death of the husband results in a great drop
of status for the widow, especially if she has no living sons. She remains in
the household of the in-laws and her lot is completely dependent upon the
behavior of these in-laws. She is called an "inauspicious thing," traditionally
made visible and unattractive by diet and clothing and can sometimes be

treated as a servant. The reform movements in India are also directed toward the improvement of the situation of widows.

RELATIONS WITH IN-LAWS IN MODERN SOCIETIES

An interesting phenomenon can be observed in literature on the modern American family, and that is the relative absence of reference to in-law relationships. There are several reasons for the decrease of attention and, by implication, of importance of the in-laws. One of the consequences of societal changes in the direction of increased complexity of scale in more modernized societies has been the decrease of intergenerational patriarchy, or the power of the male descent line over a young nuclear family.

The male was the first to be freed from the life-long control by the family line as a result of his increased dependence on education and individually acquired jobs. These trends enabled a freer selection of a spouse and nuclear residence of his family of procreation. Although the freeing of the husband from kin dependency also frees the wife from control by her in-laws, it simultaneously deprives her of the support systems they provided. This is especially true if the nuclear unit lives independently from the husband's family of orientation.

Uniquely American is the fact that most of the life of its "modern," mainly middle-class, segments is *not* built around kinship relations of either descent line (Aulette, 1994). Kin tend to be socially and geographically dispersed and unavailable for extensive contact or supports. Basically, kin relationships are developed by choice beyond this central descent line of 2-3 generations, and sometimes even within it. One indication of the last named tendency is the asymmetry of relationships with the husband's and the wife's family (Lopata, 1994). The nineteenth-century division of the world into a private sphere, under the domination of the woman, and a public sphere, the province of the man, accompanied by the decrease of responsibility of the man for the welfare of his extended family, resulted in a shift in the closeness of the nuclear unit from the male line to the female line. The ideological construction of the world into these two spheres, in reality quite artificial, has of recent decades been questioned by feminists and pulled together by the behavior of women and men (Lopata, 1993).

Let me briefly explain the shift of relational closeness from the male to the female line. Patriarchal societies demanded that the oldest male carry the responsibility for the whole family, his elderly parents, wife and unmarried (sometimes even married sons) offspring, unmarried (sometimes even married) siblings, and even kin removed by another generation, such as grandparents and grandchildren. Admittedly his wife and the other women of the family carried forth the supportive work required by this responsibility, but it was his obligation to insure that they did it (Lopata, 1990).

The mother-daughter connection was not very close in societies in which she had to leave, often with a family-impoverishing dowry, early in life and devote herself to her mother-in-law's welfare. The freeing of the nuclear unit from the male line enables the daughter and mother to develop and maintain close, life-long ties. Chodorow (1978), Rossi and Rossi (1990) and others claim that this mother-daughter tie is biologically based and results in similarities in social roles. However, they neglect the cases in which the daughter cannot build and retain such ties but must separate herself from her mother because she leaves to join the husband's family (Lopata, 1990). It is the son with whom the traditional Indian mother developed the closest relationships (Lopata, 1979, 1990) and his wife had to be subservient to her mother-in-law. The modern daughter is no longer obligated to identify with, and be totally responsible for, her mother-in-law, while the mother-daughter tie is encouraged. This shift makes the husband the outsider of the relationship of his wife and children to her parents. His emphasis upon his public life, socialized into with the help of the Protestant Ethic, results in his separation from the family of orientation and even secondary involvement in his family of procreation. Thus, he is not seen, and does not usually behave, as responsible for maintaining contact with any extended kin, even his own. His contact with his in-laws is through the wife and she has minimal obligations to her in-laws.

The exceptions to the above model appear in the descriptions of both lower- and upper-class American families. According to Ostrander (1984) upper-class women have to keep in close contact with whichever kin are responsible for, or at least have contributed to, this social status (Papanek, 1979). They cannot allow any other involvements, including status-maintaining volunteer work, to interfere with obligations to the kin network (Daniels, 1988). By the way, the network does not contain anyone who is not of equal or higher status even if biologically related.

Hareven (1978) established the fact that the processes of modernization presented in the ideal-typical model of family life do not apply to many ethnic groups. In-law relations within these communities have interesting variations (Litwak, 1960; Sussman, 1953, 1962, 1965). Mindel, Habenstein, and Wright's (1988) *Ethnic Families in America* is full of descriptions of the supports provided to all generations by in-laws, as well as consanguine relatives.

The importance of kinship relationships has also been noted in studies of African American lower-class families (Stack, 1975; Jarrett, 1990a, 1990b; McAdoo, 1981; Taylor, Chatters & Mays, 1988). Jarrett (1990b) points to a very important fact that the father's relatives may be active participants in the child's support systems even if there is no in-law relationship with the mother. Hays and Mindel (1973) compared white and black families and found the latter perceived interaction with kin as much more significant and involving a broader range of members than did the former. This included in-laws who are active in child-care and even likely to share housing at one time or another. Jackson and Berg-Cross (1988) also emphasize the importance of the mother-in-law to a young woman.

This brings us to a very interesting gap in most status attainment and intergenerational occupational mobility literature. Very few scholars consider the contributions of in-laws to a man's (certainly not to a woman's) occupation. The only place one can find references to a father-in-law bringing the son-in-law into an occupation or a job is in biographies of family dynasties or the recent books on family business (Ward, 1987; Ward & Mendoza, 1996).

Rosenblatt and his associates (1985: 174) discuss the business community's attitudes toward sons-in-law who become successors of the founder's business in the absence of sons, or absence of willing and able sons, who are the preferred inheritors:

> The American kinship system values blood relationships. Many Americans do not consider in-laws to be relatives (Schneider, 1980). When a son-in-law enters a business and assumes the role of successor or potential successor to control or ownership, some people consider that to be in some way inappropriate. The son-in-law may be suspected of being avaricious and manipulative, to have violated some cultural rule.

FEELINGS AND ATTITUDES AMONG IN-LAWS

Most American parents-in-law lack societally approved control over the younger generation, which can even remove itself from contact. However, complete lack of contact is relatively rare. The presence of mother-in-law and the infrequent father-in-law jokes indicate at least some contact and consequent tension. The jokes are usually told by the son-in-law but the daughter-in-law and mother-in-law conflict appears in the popular and some sociological literature. The gender differences can be accounted for to a major extent by the fact that the mother-in-law, especially one not involved in a career, is more likely to be in contact with the younger couple than is her husband and that she may be more apt to be seen as "interfering" in their life in the private domain (Fischer, 1983a).

The classic study of in-law relationships by Evelyn Duvall (1954) discussed both the comparative freedom of choice and the complications of relationships in a society that did not force the daughter-in-law to live with, and provide supports to, the relatives of her husband. Her title, *In-laws: Pro and Con* is indicative of the "modern" situation. Avoidance rituals are absent, but stereotypes of mothers-in-law abound and relations with them are considered more problematic than those with other in-laws, such as fathers or siblings. In contrast Duvall (1954) obtained 3,683 responses from a radio appeal for answers to "Why I think mothers-in-law are wonderful people." Recent, usually more methodologically sound, although still infrequent, studies have focused on the specifics of the relationship between the mother-in-law and the daughter-in-law.

Lucy Fischer (1983a: 394) introduces her research note on *Married Men and their Mothers* with the folk saying:

A daughter is a daughter the rest of her life;
A son is a son until he takes a wife.

Again, this is a very non-patriarchal definition of the situation, in that the daughter can remain close to her mother, while a son is not obliged to do so. In fact, Fischer found that the wife mediates the relations not only between her husband and her parents, but also and even more so once children are born, between her husband and his own mother. She concluded that even in recent times the son's physical care for his parents in the absence of a daughter is actually carried out by his wife, while he is not strongly involved in care of his in-laws. This combination can create resentment on the part of the daughter-in-law if the burden falls on her since she is not likely to be close to the husband's parents.

Fischer also reemphasized the usual assumption that mothers-in-law are more "likely to have strained relationships with daughters-in-law than with sons-in-law" (Fischer, 1983b:190). However, the mother-in-law must establish some positive relations with the son's wife if she wants to be involved with the grandchildren. She also found that, although a woman's relationship with her own mother becomes closer with the birth of her children, it increases "the ambiguity in the quasi-kin, quasi-maternal relationship between mothers-in-law and daughters-in-law" (Fischer, 1986:191). The awkwardness of the relationship can be indicated by the fact that mothers-in-law tend to give the daughter-in-law things, while the mother is more likely to perform services for her daughter. The younger woman is apt to express ambivalence over help from the in-laws and ask her mother rather than her mother-in-law for advice.

The fact that in-laws are a secondary relationship, acquired arbitrarily through the primary tie between a husband and a wife, may account for part of the problem in in-law interaction. This is complicated by the probability, especially in a society as heterogeneous as the American, that the spouses come from different backgrounds, accentuated in their parents' generation, which may clash over ritualistic or day-by-day life styles. Of course, popular culture emphasizes the alleged feeling of all parents that the person the offspring marries is never good enough. Certainly the parents-in-law are often seen as below the self in social status and knowledge of what is good for the grandchildren.

As in all social interaction, many factors influence the quality of the relationships among in-laws (Goetting, 1990). Marotz-Baden and Cowan (1987) found proximity contributing to conflict and stress, especially if there is a business or secondary relationship involved. Their study focused on farm and ranch families who were living and farming together. Conflict among the cohabitors was most frequent between the mother- and the daughter-in-law and focused on child rearing values and opinions. Interestingly enough, twice as many mothers- as daughters-in-law reported no problems at all (p. 387). Of course, they are more apt to have greater power in the relationship than do the younger women.

The possibility that in-law relationships can have a forced, or at least not fully voluntary, quality is indicated by the frequency with which they wither after divorce and widowhood. This was definitely the case with American urban widows (Lopata, 1973, 1979). In-laws might be present and provide some support around the time of the death and funeral, but most widows do not consider them as supportive of themselves and even of the children in later times. The one exception are families with definite financial or service benefits and possibilities of inheritance (Lopata, 1979).

Divorce is especially apt to end or weaken the relationships between in-laws of even three generations. The divorcing husband and wife are likely to require loyalty from their own kin and to interpret continued contact with the other spouse as betrayal, or at least unfavorably. A major problem in this situation is usually the grandparent-grandchildren interaction. Active grandparents can become deeply disturbed over a break in their contact with the grandchildren, to the extent of even organizing to obtain formal rights of visitation (Johnson, 1988, 1989; Lager, 1977). This is certainly different from the traditional situation in which, for example, the divorcing wife had to leave her children with the husband's family if she left (Bohannan, 1963) and her family of orientation never did have rights over them. Johnson (1988) covers the problems of grandparents in divorcing families in her *Ex Familia*, explaining that the norms that regulate the relationships are vague. Of course, the responses to separation and divorce depend to a great extent on the "styles of grandparenting." Many grandparents are simply too socially and emotionally distant from the grandchildren to be strongly affected by a break in contact. The actions of the middle generation have obvious consequences on what is possible in these relationships and in-laws of the custodial parent are less likely to be able to continue active grandparenting.

This is particularly true in case of remarriage by either or both of the ex-partners:

[D]ivorce entails major alterations in the use of social and other resources of the local kin network. Divorced and remarried women are unlikely to contact or receive help from their former spouse's kindred. Remarried women are, however, integrated into the kin network of their present spouse's kindred, while the kin networks of the divorced are imbalanced. (Anspach, 1976, p. 329)

CONCLUSIONS

Gubrium and Holstein (1990) asked, "What is family?" This is certainly a complicated question when in-laws are considered. These relations are created by marriage, not just of the self, but also of others, as in the case of the marriage of one's children. In-laws can be acquired at any stage of the life course through no choice of one's own, or as an after effect of another choice. Of course, many other family relations are entered into involuntarily, i.e., they are ascribed, not achieved, even in an achievement-oriented society. This is true of one's parents and their consanguine kin. The choice is on the part of the parents who must decide to enter the roles of mother and father through their own action, by "natural birth" and its modern variations or by adoption. The biological fact of reproduction does not, however, guarantee the social role, entrance into which must be recognized by the social person and members of the social circle (Lopata, 1994). And, it is possible to renounce the role, as when adopting parents reject the child, or parents give up a biological offspring to others.

In-law relations, however, can be entered into as active social roles through the same process of self and other identification. It is thus important to recognize that a family relationship is not an automatic one, but involves entrance into appropriate social roles with those that the law recognizes as connected through the marriage of other people. In fact, the presence of fictive in-law relationships indicates that the law is even an unnecessary precondition. What remains is the social role itself: the set of relations between the social person who declares her/himself a mother- father- daughter- sister- brother- grandparent- grandchild- aunt- uncle- cousin- and so forth in-law, and obtains the cooperation of a social circle, including the "beneficiary" of the relation and all the assisting segments (Lopata, 1971; Lopata, Miller, & Barnewolt, 1986). Thus, according to my definition, a family is a group of people entered into family relationships by entering the appropriate social roles.

Changes in all kinds of human relationships raise many questions as to in-laws. How do the two sets of in-laws, from the husband and wife, relate to the couple? What factors affect the degree of influence or power each can exert? How does the younger generation relate upwards to the parents-in-law and collateral in-laws? What, if any, are the differences in the expected closeness in relationships between brothers and their wives versus sisters and their husbands? What happens to in-law relationships after divorce and how does the connection to the ex-in-law affect grandparent-grandchild interaction? To what extent are similar relations extended to cohabitors who are not married? What happens to "in-lawship" when such a couple has children to whom the members of the older generation are grandparents?

REFERENCES

Anspach, D. (1976). Kinship and divorce. *Journal of Marriage and the Family, 38*, 323-330.

Aulette, J. R. (1994). *Changing families*. Belmont, CA: Wadsworth.

Barnes, D. R. (1987). Wives and widows in China. In H. Z. Lopata (Ed.), *Widows: The Middle East, Asia and the Pacific* (pp. 194-216). Durham, NC: Duke University Press.

Bhatia, S. et al. (1987). High risk suicide factors across cultures. *International Journal of Social Psychiatry, 33*, 226-236.

Bohannan, P. J. (1963). *Social Anthropology*. New York: Holt, Rinehart and Winston.

Chodorow, N. (1978). *The reproduction of mothering: Psychoanalysis and the sociology of gender*. Berkeley: University of California Press.

Daniels, A. (1988). *Invisible careers: Women community leaders in the volunteer world*. Chicago: University of Chicago Press.

Duvall, E. (1954). *In-laws: Pro and con*. New York: Association Press.

Eichler, M. (1973). Women as personal dependents. In M. Stephenson (Ed.), *Women in Canada* (pp. 36-55). Toronto: New Press.

Fischer, L. (1983a). Married men and their mothers. *Journal of Comparative Family Studies, 14*, 394-402.

Fischer, L. (1983b). Mothers and mothers-in-law. *Journal of Marriage and the Family, 14*, 187-192.

Fischer, L. (1986). *Linked lives: Adult daughters and their mothers*. New York: Harper and Row.

Goetting, A. (1990). Patterns of support among in-laws in the United States: A review of research. *Journal of Family Issues, 11*, 67-90.

Gubrium, J., & Holstein, J. (1990). *What is Family?: An ethnomethodoligical approach*. Mountain View, CA: Mayfield.

Hareven, T. K. (1978). The dynamics of kin in an industrial community. In J. Demos & S. Boocock (Eds.), *Turning Points* (pp. 151-181). Chicago: University of Chicago Press.

Hays, W. C., & Mindel, C. H. (1973). Extended kinship relations in black and white families. *Journal of Marriage and the Family, 35*, 51-57.

Jackson, J., & Berg-Cross, L. (1988). Extending the extended family: The mother-in-law and daughter-in-law relationship of Black women. *Family Relations, 37*(3), 293-297.

Jarrett, R. (1990a). *A comparative examination of socialization patterns among low-*

income African-Americans, Chicanos and Puerto Ricans and Whites: A Review of the ethnographic literature. Report to the Social Science Research Council.

Jarrett, R. (1990b). Family life and socialization patterns among low-income black women: An ethnographic exploration. Report to the Spencer Foundation.

Johnson, C. L. (1988). Ex familia: grandparents, parents, and children adjust to divorce. New Brunswick, Rutgers University Press.

Johnson, C. L. (1989). In-law relationships in the American kinship system: The impact of divorce and remarriage. American Ethnologist, 16, 87-99.

Khan, M. Z., & Rav, R. 1984. Dowry death. Indian Journal of Social Work, 45, 303-315.

Lager, E. (1977). Parents-in-law: Failure and divorce in a second chance family. Journal of Marriage and Family Counseling, 3, 19-23.

Litwak, E. (1960). Geographical mobility and extended family cohesion. American Sociological Review, 25, 385-394.

Lopata, H. Z. (1971). Occupation: Housewife. New York: Oxford University Press.

Lopata, H. Z. (1973). Widowhood in an American city. Cambridge, MA: Schenkman.

Lopata, H. Z. (1979). Women as widows: Support systems. New York: Elsevier.

Lopata, H. Z. (1990). Which child? The consequences of social development on the support systems of widows. In B. Hess & E. Markson, (Eds.), Growing old in America (pp. 39-49). New Brunswick, NJ: Transaction.

Lopata, H. Z. (1993). The interweave of public and private: Women's challenge to American society. Journal of Marriage and the Family, 55, 220-235.

Lopata, H. Z. (1994). Circles and Settings: Role changes of American women. Philadelphia: Temple University Press.

Lopata, H. Z., Miller, C. A., & Barnewolt, D. (1986). City women in America. New York: Praeger.

Marotz-Baden, R., & Cowan, D. (1987). Mothers-in-law and daughters-in-law: The effects of proximity on conflict and stress. Family Relations, 36, 385-390.

McAdoo, H. P. (1981). Black families. Beverly Hills, CA: Sage.

Mindel, C., Habenstein, R. W., & Wright, R., Jr. (1988). Ethnic families in America (3rd ed.). New York: Elsevier.

Murdock, G. (1949). Social structure. New York: Macmillan.

Ostrander, S. (1984). Women of the upper class. Philadelphia: Temple University Press. The Oxford universal dictionary (1995). Oxford: At the Clarendon Press.

Papanek, H. (1979). Family status production: The 'work' and 'non-work' of women. Signs, 4, 775-781.

Parasuraman, S. (1986). Migration and its effect on the family. Indian Journal of Social Work, 47, 1-14.

Pillai, T. V. (1982). Prostitution in India. Indian Journal of Social Work, 43, 313-320.

Rosenblatt, P. C. et al., (1985). The family in business. San Francisco: Jossey-Bass.

Rossi, A. & Rossi, P. (1990). Of human bonding: Parent-child relations across the life course. New York: Aldine/de Guyter.

Stack, C. (1975). All our kin. New York: Harper & Row.

Sussman, M. B. (1953). The help patterns in the middle class family. American Sociological Review, 18, 22-28.

Sussman, M. B. (1962). The Isolated Nuclear Family: Fact or Fiction. In R. Winch

(Ed.), *Selected Studies in Marriage and the Family* (pp. 49-57). New York: Holt Rinehart & Winston.

Sussman, M. B. (1965). Relationships of Adult Children with their Parents in the United States. In E. Shanas & G. Streib (Eds.), *Social Structure and the Family: Generational Relations* (pp. 62-72). Englewood Cliffs, NJ: Prentice-Hall.

Taylor, R. J., Chatters, L., & Mays, L. (1988). Parents, children, siblings, in-laws and non-kin as sources of emergency assistance to Black Americans. *Family Relations, 37*, 298-304.

Ward, J. (1987). *Keeping Family Business Healthy*. San Francisco, CA: Jossey Bass.

Ward, J., & Mendoza, D. (1966). Work in Family Business. In H. Z. Lopata & A. Figert (Eds.), *Current Research in Occupations and Professions: Getting Down to Business* (pp. 167-188). Greenwich, CT: JAI Press.

Wolfram, S. (1987). *In-Laws and Outlaws: Kinship and Marriage in England*. New York: St. Martin's Press.

Negotiating Family:
The Interface Between Family
and Support Groups

Ruth Flexman
Debra L. Berke
Barbara H. Settles

INTRODUCTION

Families live in an elaborate network of interacting ties of varying complexity and strength with a broad array of other individuals, families, and larger social collectives (Milardo, 1988). One of the new social collectives that has expanded dramatically in the recent past is the gathering of individuals who share a common problem or concern in support groups. The relationships between families and support groups will be explored in this paper, with an important purpose being to examine how and where exchanges occur between these two social entities.

Social support as a broader system of extra-familial ties has been widely studied. Significant research attention has documented that the presence of a strong social support system can reduce stress (Cobb, 1976; Dean & Lin, 1977; De Araujo, Van Arsdel, Holmes & Dudley, 1973; Nuckolls, Cassel & Kaplan, 1972; Williams, 1985), increase life satisfaction (Lowenthal & Haven, 1968), and increase one's sense of well-being (Leveton, Griffin & Douglas, 1979; Shumaker & Brownell, 1984). Lack of social support has been

---

Ruth Flexman is affiliated with University of Delaware, Newark, DE 19716.

Debra L. Berke is affiliated with Messiah College, Grantham, PA.

Barbara H. Settles is affiliated with Department of Individual and Family Studies, University of Delaware, Newark, DE 19716.

[Haworth co-indexing entry note]: "Negotiating Family: The Interface Between Family and Support Groups." Flexman, Ruth, Debra L. Berke, and Barbara H. Settles. Co-published simultaneously in *Marriage & Family Review* (The Haworth Press, Inc.) Vol. 28, No. 3/4, 1999, pp. 173-190; and: *Concepts and Definitions of Family for the 21st Century* (ed: Barbara H. Settles et al.) The Haworth Press, Inc., 1999, pp. 173-190. Single or multiple copies of this article are available for a fee from The Haworth Document Delivery Service [1-800-342-9678, 9:00 a.m. - 5:00 p.m. (EST). E-mail address: getinfo@haworthpressinc.com].

linked to vulnerability, health disorders, suicide, emotional and social isolation, as well as loneliness (Weiss, 1973; Williams, 1985). Social support has been characterized as providing five different support functions: financial, physical, emotional, advice/guidance, and socializing (Berke, 1991, adapted from Barrera & Ainley, 1983).

Traditionally, social support in times of crisis or loss was provided within the family setting. Most families had contact with few social institutions outside of churches and schools. The local family doctor or healer was the sole provider of medical care and when problems or losses occurred, options and expectations for dealing with these issues were minimal.

Subsequently, however, the nature of support systems has changed. Few people now remain close to their places of birth throughout their life spans. Thus, life-long neighbors and kin may not be available to provide the primary sources of support. Now many different organizations offer services to families; the family doctor, for example, orchestrates a spectrum of referrals to numerous diagnostic and treatment options and the expectations for successful treatment have expanded dramatically with advances in technology. As a result, the family is faced with major changes in responsibility for participation in these decisions (Settles, 1987). Today's adult children may be called upon to make end-of-life medical decisions on behalf of their parents concerning treatment alternatives.

Increasing geographical distance and technological advances in treatment have influenced the decision-making and support functions within the family structure. Support and information may not be adequately provided by the family system at this point in history due to such developments as industrialization, the decreased size of family kinship systems, and the decline of informal service exchange within the community (Caplan & Killilea, 1976; Gartner & Reissman, 1977; Katz, 1981; Katz & Bender, 1976; Lieberman & Borman, 1979). Changes in family structure and increased medical and service technology may further reduce the effectiveness of support. Individuals may receive less physical and emotional support from distant family members, yet they may need more information and support for making choices that are intelligent, educated, and compassionate.

In this situation the numbers and types of support groups have expanded dramatically to address this concern by providing both the needed information and emotional support. Support groups have been defined by Katz and Bender (1976) as consisting of people gathering together for a treatment or to accomplish a specific purpose. Today, there are literally thousands of groups in the United States designed to help their members with hundreds of distinctive types of problems (Katz, 1981; Lieberman & Borman, 1979). Such groups include, for example, caregivers of patients with Alzheimer's (Gonyea, 1989), individuals who have amyotropic lateral sclerosis (Leach, 1990), single-parent mothers (Bienstock & Videka, 1989), mothers of infants with disabilities (Krauss, Upshur, Shonkoff & Hauser, 1993), individuals who test HIV positive (Greene, McVinney & Adams, 1993), those experiencing bereavement (Levy & Derby, 1992), families adopting children with developmental disabilities (Marcenko & Smith, 1991), and children of cancer patients (Call, 1990), to list just a few. In fact, the popularity of support groups might indicate that these groups are a valuable and needed resource that now represent a broad spectrum of the population that exists in response to a wide variety of afflictions. Moreover, family support efforts appear to be supplemented by the unique sharing of experiences of people who have "been there."

Although past research has focused on support systems within families and on the dynamics and functions within support groups, current scholarship has focused little attention on the interface between family microsystems and support groups when some form of mediation occurs. Two aspects of these issues will be explored initially. First an overview of the family as a microsystem, with its own definitions, boundary descriptions and illustrations of functions will be described. Subsequently, the support group as a microsystem will be described in similar terms, through such concepts as definitions, boundary limits, membership descriptions, and characterizing functions.

Following these descriptions a dynamic model is proposed to illustrate the relationship between the systems, the interface between the family and support groups as well as boundary differences that function to differentiate between the separate systems.

FAMILY AS A MICROSYSTEM

Families function as a microsystem that relates to other systems in a network of interacting ties. The family unit is comprised of family members that may appear to be a straightforward description of the boundaries of this system, but, in fact, membership in a family depends on the particular definition of a family.

Definition of Family

Traditional definitions of family have included structural dimensions, functional dimensions, or aspects of both dimensions, while other attempts to define a family include that of a group of people closely related by blood, marriage, or adoption (Zimmerman, 1988). Bane (1976) defines the family, for example, as special relational ties that reflect the need of all individuals for stability, continuity, and unconditional affection in their lives. Beutler and Burr (1989) refer to the family realm as a complex set of affect, development,

, rules, ethics, patterns, relationships, aspirations, values, and heri-
_ge. Other definitions include:

a. a group whose members who love and care for one another (Footlick,
   1989);
b. two or more persons who are related by mutual expectations of emotional and material support, regardless of their living arrangements.
   The family-like behaviors of these individuals convey mutual responsibility, intimacy and care on a continuing basis (Burant, 1989);
c. two or more persons "in a committed relationship from which they derive
   a sense of identity as a family" (Chilman, Cox, & Nunnally, 1988: xx);
d. any ongoing social arrangement in which persons care about each other
   and are committed to one another so that their basic psychological, social, physical, and economic needs can be met (Zimmerman, 1988);
   and,
e. cohabitating groups of some duration that are composed of persons in
   intimate relations which are based in biology, law, custom, choice, and
   usually in economic dependence (Aldous & Dumon, 1990).

Although family scholars have agreed that how family is defined is extremely important, they have not reached a consensus on the issues of "what
family is" even "if family" should be defined (see articles by Bernardes,
Holstein & Gubrium, Jurich & Johnson, Levin, Settles, and Trost, in this
volume).

Family Boundaries

The location and permeability of the boundaries between families and the
support groups are of interest in understanding how families relate to other
entities. When the family is defined based on structural attributes such as
marriage or birth, the concept of boundaries seems simple to grasp. However,
when functional aspects such as love and caring are considered, who is
family and who is outside family membership are more complex. Families
may create their own members as needed (Settles, 1987) to the extent that
enduring relationships with others are formed having mutual expectations.

Support Functions Families Provide

Support functions are "actions that others perform when they render assistance to a focal person" (Barrera, 1986:417), with family support systems
providing mutually beneficial, reciprocal support (Ramey, 1988). Within the
family the need for social support endures throughout life, but the particular

requirements for sources and types of social support vary with personal and situational characteristics, life cycle stage, or with life transitions or events (Blieszner, 1988). Social support remains important in mid-life normative transitions as adults confront the beginnings of physical declines (Johnson, 1988), or when they provide care for an elderly parent (Gibeau, 1986). Particular experiences also may evoke new needs and new sources of support (Blieszner, 1988). An unexpected illness or divorce, for example, may require new sources of assistance such as a support group either in addition to, or instead of, the family.

SUPPORT GROUPS AS A MICROSYSTEM

The support group functions as a microsystem that is influenced by and influencing those gathered around a common cause. Like a family, support groups differ by definition, membership, and boundary characteristics.

Definition of Support Group

Ramey (1988) has made a distinction between family support systems and non-traditional support groups. Family members provide mutually beneficial, reciprocal support in family support systems, whereas in non-traditional support groups assistance comes from outside the family. Central issues or common experiences are particularly important for drawing members together for mutual aid in support groups. Support groups can resemble families: that is, they are small face-to-face groups that mimic family-like relationships and can provide emotional support as a primary group (Bauman, Gervey & Siegel, 1992). Support groups may establish specific roles for their members, with each member having expected obligations and reciprocal behaviors towards other members (Hartley, 1988). In contrast to families as ongoing systems, support groups differ by being "small, voluntary groups designed to provide their members with support, encouragement, and a nonjudgmental, safe atmosphere in which to voice problems and concerns as well as joys and triumphs" (Rubel, 1984:382). Moreover, relationships in support groups are focused on the purpose for interaction, rather than developing into multidimensional relationships.

The terms support group, self-help group, and mutual aid group appear to be used interchangeably in much of the literature, perhaps because there is considerable overlap in practice. Theoretically, each support group has a different structure, a varied set of goals and procedures, and distinctive policies concerning the role of professionals and professional organizations (Enright, Butterfield & Berkowitz, 1985; Levy, 1982).

Boundaries of Support Groups

Froland, Pancoast, Chapman and Kimboko (1981) differentiate between "embedded" and "created" networks. While embedded networks are based on kinship, residential proximity, or organizational relationships, created networks are fostered to assist people with a similar problem or need. An interest in participation is often the only requirement for belonging to a support group. People who face specific types of problems or circumstances often feel, with good reason, that most people cannot understand what they are experiencing. These individuals often claim to have a special kind of understanding and mutuality shared only by persons who have gone through the same event or situation (George, 1987, p. 319).

Membership

Demographic factors have been demonstrated to influence who chooses to become members of support groups. The boundaries of support groups, therefore, are not only related to the particular circumstance, but also to gender, class, education, and income levels.

Research on support group participation is consistent with findings from research on voluntary associations in general. People who are middle or upper class, well educated and have higher than average incomes are more likely than lower-middle or working-class individuals to participate in mutual aid or meetings (Bond & Daiter, 1979; Borman, 1982; Durman, 1976; Edwards, Hensman, Hawker & Williamson, 1966; Fried, 1976; Lieberman & Borman, 1979; McAfee, 1952; Wheat & Lieber, 1979). Women are more likely than men to make use of resources (Chesler, Barbarin & Lebo-Stein, 1984; Hinrichsen, Revenson & Shinn, 1985; Levy, 1976; Videka-Sherman, 1982) and the typical caregiver's support group is composed predominantly of white, middle-class females, ages 40-65, who are related to the person needing care (Toseland & Rossiter, 1989). This limited participation, however, is not universal (Koroloff & Friesen, 1991). Knight, Wollert, Levy, Frame and Padgett (1980) and Telleen, Herzog and Kilbane (1989) provide evidence that group participation can encompass a wider membership than is generally assumed.

Sharing a central problem defines a person's membership status in a support group despite many individual differences in background. A peer in a group has a commonality or mutuality with others (Katz, 1970). In her study of Al-Anon, for example, Ablon (1974) found that many individuals had come to Al-Anon thinking that they alone had suffered 'unique' experiences. Of utmost importance in their experience, in turn, was recognizing the universality of these problems and finding a safe arena in which to talk about their feelings and modes of handling the problems.

Functions of Support Groups

Three issues must be addressed for a support group's sense of integrity to be defined: (1) the purpose of the group, (2) the group membership, and (3) the effectiveness of the group in achieving its purpose (Ramey, 1988). Support groups serve to permit people who share common concerns to meet one another, seek appropriate solutions for their problems, and form supportive relationships (George, 1987). Regardless of the particular problem or issue of concern, support groups tend to share three common generic goals (Lieberman & Borman, 1979). These goals are: (1) to educate participants about the nature of the problem and the most effective methods of managing or alleviating the problem; (2) to provide members with an opportunity to share their feelings with others who have had similar experiences; and (3) to provide participants with opportunities to develop ongoing relationships with others who are socially similar and share common interests.

Toseland and Rossiter (1989) examine a number of functions that support groups provide. Group interventions to support family caregivers have the potential to prevent stressors from overwhelming caregivers by: providing a much-needed respite from caregiving; reducing isolation and loneliness; providing an opportunity to share feelings and experiences in a supportive environment with peers who share similar concerns; providing caregivers with support, understanding, and affirmation; validating thoughts and feelings about caregiving; universalizing and normalizing caregivers' experiences; and assuring caregivers that they are playing a vital role in providing care. Providing information is another function of support groups: educating caregivers about the effects of chronic disabilities; informing them about community resources; and encouraging a mutual sharing of information about effective coping strategies. Additional executive functions include: helping caregivers to identify and examine problems and concerns as well as using systematic problem-solving procedures to resolve specific concerns (Toseland & Rossiter, 1989).

Different presenting problems necessitate support groups with differing agendas, styles and sequences. Parents of children with special health-care needs reported that support groups were most helpful when their child was better, at diagnosis, and at times of family crisis. Specific aspects of the group they liked best were the support received from the group and the information received about resources and their child's illness or disability (Smith, Gabard, Dale & Drucker, 1994). The type of problems affect whether support is needed and helpful for either a brief or more extended period of time. Lengthy support is necessary, for example, in the case of Alzheimer's Disease, which progresses over a number of years, but only for a relatively short, intense time of grieving when such an event as death through SIDS (Sudden Infant Death Syndrome) occurs. Caregivers and patients may seek different things from groups, such as information from experts or contact with other Amyotropic lateral sclerosis (ALS) patients (Leach, 1990).

Support groups allow their members to have a measure of control over how they will relate to the group. This self-control applies to the information and ideas to which they are exposed during the group process. Individuals may choose the level of involvement and the amount of self-disclosure that matches their comfort level, with boundaries being negotiated by both the person and the group. In addition, the helper roles that each person may play in the group may be important in expanding the self efficacy and learning of the individual (Ramsey, 1992).

THEORETICAL PARADIGM

The beneficial impact of support groups occurs by interfacing with the family system. Consequently, how families and support groups interface is vitally important to understanding the success of support groups. Identifying the definitions and boundary lines of family and support group microsystems specifies what is included and excluded from the individual systems. The characteristics of this interface can be clarified by using a model that describes the process of mediating between systems of family and support groups.

A theoretical perspective also is needed to aid in examining and analyzing the support group-familial interface. An ecological paradigm (Maton, 1994) provides a useful perspective for examining the interrelationships between families and support groups. This interface between families and support groups is complex and can be described as "more a tapestry than a thread" (Vaux & Athanassopulou, 1987, p. 548). Although some distinctions or patterns are clear, interrelationships exist that vary with individuals, with families, and with support groups. This ecological paradigm has several assumptions which make it useful for studying the complexity of the interface between family and support group:

1. social phenomena occur within and are shaped by a complex, interrelated network of factors that span multiple variable domains and levels of analysis; and
2. there are multiple and reciprocal pathways of influence among variables.

The proposed paradigm suggests how to examine this interface by studying the interface between the family setting and the support group in which the precipitating event or circumstance occurs. Moreover, to address the point of interface between these distinct microsystems, it is first necessary to consider the differentiating characteristics of the family and the support group.

Interface Between Families and Support Groups

How do the two microsystems, families and support groups, interact and how do connections between these two systems operate? What is the relationship between the family and inclusion in a particular support group? The following figure is designed to illustrate the relationships between families and support groups (see Figure 1).

In the diagram, the boundaries around the family as well as the support group are shown by broken lines to indicate both microsystems' permeability which allows inputs and outputs from one system to another. The arrow designates the reciprocity of this process, while the X indicates the contact person(s), individual(s) and/or family members, who mediate relationships between the two systems. This mediator role is the key aspect of relationships between the two microsystems.

Boundary Differences Between Families and Support Groups

Both the family and support group microsystems have boundaries, but family boundaries are different than those around support groups for a variety of reasons. Table 1 compares boundary differences between the family and support groups along the dimensions of definition, uniqueness, intimacy, trust and disclosure, and information gathering and exchange.

It is necessary to examine the differences in the characteristics of boundaries for support groups and families to gain an understanding of the structure and dynamics of the interface between them. The family boundaries as defined by the support group may change over time as the family structure is modified by life transitions. Specific family members included and how many are involved in a support group differ among support groups. For example, in the groups that have been created to help alcoholics and their families, spouses and children are traditionally served separately as individuals and only rarely are brought together as family groups. In contrast, child-

FIGURE 1. Relationship between the family and the support group.

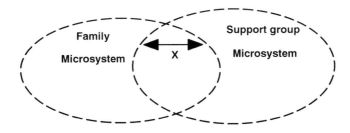

TABLE 1. Boundary differences between families and support groups.

	FAMILY	SUPPORT GROUPS
Definition	May be structurally or functionally defined.	Related by need precipitated by common stressful experience.
Uniqueness	Perceive boundaries which define their situation as unusual.	Boundaries around support group enclose people sharing common knowledge of "how it is."
Intimacy trust vs. disclosure	Boundaries form around the family unit to protect family secrets; stress may isolate family.	Individual boundaries become permeable with assumed intimacy based on shared common experiences.
Information gathering	Boundaries are limited to family experiences and what information a family can access.	Boundaries for information access are broadened to include real life experiences and the cumulative information assembled by group members.

hood disease and handicapped groups, such as juvenile diabetes, cystic fibrosis, and muscular dystrophy, frequently serve more of the whole family (including siblings) in their meetings and programs. Moreover, the primary caregiver in support groups for Alzheimer's patients frequently attends the group both without other family members or the patient. The support group, therefore, serves as a respite for the caregiver. Distance and confidentiality from the family, nearby neighbors, and community may be treasured parts of the group process.

The boundaries surrounding support groups are defined by the sharing of a common situation. Support groups have arisen around specific concerns and not generic needs of families for a supportive community and social ties. Boundary concerns and rapport are centered on understanding a specific unmet need rather than a general understanding of friendship and intimate ties. The intimacy of the support or group is achieved not by sharing a broad array of interests and personal information, but by the recognition of the impact of some trauma, challenge or loss upon the person and/or family. The strength and tenacity of the group ties are no doubt partially related to the life course trajectory of the problem addressed and may require moving from one group to a related one as needs change. Cancer support groups may lead to either a survivors' or a grief group. The appeal of these groups may depend on both personality and process preferences of those in need of support.

To further explore these relationships between the two systems and their interface, boundary exchanges between the family and the support group will be discussed using the following characteristics. Caplan (1976) identified supportive functions of the family that have common characteristics attributed to support groups: (1) collectors and disseminators of information about the world; (2) a feed-back guidance system; (3) sources of ideology; (4) guides and mediators in problem-solving; (5) sources of practical service and concrete aid; (6) a haven for rest and recuperation; (7) reference groups; (8) a source and validator of identity; and, (9) a contributor to emotional mastery. Examples are drawn from support groups that the authors have assisted.

Collectors and Disseminators of Information About the World

The support group offers the setting in which a family member can receive aid in collecting information to address the problem or concern. The issue then crosses over the family boundary into the support group. As a participant in the support group, the member acts both as disseminator and collector of information. When he or she returns to the family setting, the level of sharing the information gained may be mediated by the individual. For example, the wife of a man who has just been diagnosed with diabetes goes to a support group. She hears how other families are adapting to eating and living patterns to conform to the restricted diet and need for exercise of the diabetic. Recipes may be offered. Reading labels and other practical aspects of selecting foods may be part of the discussion. With her expanded knowledge of shopping and food preparation, she can select and prepare food appropriate for her husband's condition and her view of his preferences.

This example illustrates the flow of information back and forth between systems via the attending family member or mediator. As the mediator, the participant takes the problem from the family to the support group where she receives information and support. She then returns to the family system with renewed energy and fresh information to address the presenting problem. She then returns to the support group where she can share information and provide inspiration for helping others with similar issues.

A Feedback Guidance System

Although the implementation of chosen alternatives occurs within the family setting, the exploration of alternatives often occurs within the support group setting. A participant may offer a number of possible alternatives and even be aided by other members in generating possibilities. The group can also participate in exploring possible outcomes for different alternatives based on technical information or personal experience.

A group for abused women may focus on both the emotional and practical aspects of leaving an abusive husband. Subsequently, the group may help their peer victim identify the cycles in their relationships that lead to abuse. They may provide information about alternatives such as how to find a place to live, how to escape safely if they fear bodily harm, how to care for the children, or how to deal with friends and relatives. Because fear of both leaving and staying can paralyze a woman, the process of exploring alternatives in the safety of the group allows her to face her situation and assess alternatives, which she may or may not implement in her familial situation.

Sources of Ideology and Guides and Mediators in Problem Solving

The support group may serve as a guide for problem solving and as an indirect mediator of the family system. Group members may share experiences for coping with similar problems. These shared experiences not only expand the scope of possible alternatives, but also generalize the problems in a manner that allows alternatives to be viewed more objectively. Thus, process occurs, both through expanded information and depersonalization of the problem.

The mother of an only child attended a support group for parents. Her household was in a state of turmoil because her husband was constantly berating their 10-year-old son for his immature behavior and B average in school. By attending her support group, however, she found that other boys behaved similarly to her son. She also found that unreasonable expectations of children are common and that parents frequently disagree about how to manage their children's behavior. The group served as a source of mediation for her son. She brought back into the family a more appropriate view of normal behavior and ideas for helping her husband enjoy different stages of their son's development.

Sources of Practical Service and Concrete Aid

Support groups differ widely in the amount of practical service and concrete aid considered to be appropriate roles for the participants. Some individual members may link systems and exchange aid bilaterally. The group, as a whole, may link the family to community resources that offer concrete services. Thus, while connections may occur in the support group context, the actual service rendered occurs in the family setting. Concrete aid generally occurs informally between members of the support group, rather than as part of a planned program. Two mothers of handicapped children agree to learn about caring for each other's child and exchange sitting services. Information may also be shared about services such as day care that can be purchased.

A Haven for Rest and Recuperation. The support group meeting can provide a brief rest from caregiving or other stress by associating with others who understand the dilemmas without making demands for ongoing relationships or instrumental assistance. Support groups affirm the need for rest and recuperation and offer ideas for achieving "time for one's self." Feelings may be shared which the participant may have been unwilling or unable to reveal to the family. Resources for respite care may also be identified.

Emotional support, a major function of mutual aid groups, offers recuperative and restorative powers. Comments like "I don't know how I would have made it through without knowing that I could come back and get recharged" are common affirmations at group meetings. The recuperative forces can extend beyond the boundaries of the support group.

Reference Groups. Support groups function to prevent feelings of alienation and isolation by gathering people together with like problems. This new reference group decreases the feelings of shame and blame. Through this created network, members can compare their behaviors with those of others in similar situations and learn alternative methods of handling situations. This safe comparison promotes acknowledging and modifying behaviors that result from lack of control or inappropriate choices. For example, parents in an abuse prevention support group may learn that shaking a small child is unacceptable behavior resulting from their loss of control and why it is dangerous. They are offered safer outlets for anger and nonviolent alternatives for modifying the unacceptable behaviors of their children.

Admitting that a spouse has been diagnosed with Alzheimer's Disease brings sadness from loss to the marital relationship as well as to other family and social relationships. The patient's behaviors may be embarrassing, with the victim as well as the spouse trying to deny or at least hide the affliction. Joining a support group acknowledges the reality of the diagnosis and offers a setting where honesty can prevail. Information about the disease and techniques for assisting the spouse can alleviate the situation in the home setting. How public the admission becomes accepted depends on the choices of the individuals and the definition of the situation. For example, many families were supported in admitting their own problems when the Reagan family publicized the fact that former President Ronald Reagan had been diagnosed with Alzheimer's Disease. Caregivers for Alzheimer's victims cannot hope for recovery, but can learn that they are not alone and gain a new perspective on their situation. Boss (1993, p. 164) notes that families "can at least be in charge of their definitions of the situation."

A Source and Validation of Identity. Joining a support group requires an admission and identification with a problem or issue. Some participants join a support group but are very selective in whom they tell about joining this group. Parents may not tell children that they attend a parenting group or older relatives that they attend a caregiver group. The validation of identity through membership occurs within the support group, but such identification may not extend within the family boundary.

A Contributor to Emotional Mastery. Emotional mastery is practiced within the family setting but the resources of information, modeling, developing alternatives, consoling and cheerleading occur within the support group setting. Typical comments at a support meeting include "I am at my wit's end. I just don't know if I can go on. I don't know what to do." Such comments express the depression and discouragement felt by individuals who are emotionally distraught and out of control.

Members of a support group can assist by listening to feelings, assess the depth of despair, and determine whether professional help is needed. They can aid their peers in gaining a renewed sense of personal control and of hope. The power of feeling understood and supported brings strength for coping into the afflicted situation.

CONCLUSION

Support groups are a relatively new phenomenon for providing emotional support and information that was once provided by families. The dramatic increase in the numbers of groups indicates the importance of these microsystems in relationship to other systems. The definition of family from a functional perspective may be useful to identify which family member or members may be included in a support group, but few support groups attempt to address the family as a whole. Because most support groups focus on a single dimension based on a common experience, they are limited to providing individual emotional support and information-giving aspects of social support. The family continues to struggle with the financial and physical supports. As networks that are created rather than embedded, support groups coexist with primary or family groups. For interactions to occur, a contact must be made through individuals who, as mediators, move between the two microsystems.

Families and support groups both exist as microsystems. Considering the functions of individual systems is a necessary prerequisite for understanding the dynamics of the interface between respective boundaries. The flow of information crosses boundaries depending upon what the mediator chooses to share between the systems. A mediator operating from an empowered position, such as a mother with a handicapped child, may initiate action within the family setting. The mediator in a powerless position, such as an abused spouse, may receive assistance from the group in setting boundaries within which they can control their level of engagement.

The interface between family and support groups becomes increasingly important with the growth in the function and number of support groups. Support groups have become a part of various therapeutic and treatment regimens in both physical and mental health. They are frequently recommended for help in coping with stressful events and may be mandated even in such areas as drug and spousal abuse situations.

The exploration of family functions as related to the support group functions illustrates the dynamic exchanges between these two systems. The model presented in this paper described the key dynamic in the effectiveness of support groups in assisting families–the interaction at the boundaries between these two systems. This interaction makes explicit and clarifies the highly significant role of individuals who mediate as members of both systems.

REFERENCES

Ablon, J. (1974). Al-Anon family groups. *American Journal of Psychotherapy, 28*, 30-45.

Aldous, J., & Dumon, W. (1990). Family policy in the 1980s: Controversy and consensus. *Journal of Marriage and the Family, 52*, 1136-1152.

Bane, M. (1976). *Here to stay: American families in the twentieth century.* New York: Basic Books.

Barrera, M. (1986). Distinctions between social support concepts, measures, and models. *American Journal of Community Psychology, 14*, 413-445.

Barrera, M., & Ainlay, S. (1983). The structure of social support: A conceptual and empirical analysis. *Journal of Community Psychology, 11*, 133-143.

Bauman, L., Gervey, R., & Siegel, K. (1992). Factors associated with cancer patients' participation in support groups. *Journal of Psychosocial Oncology, 10*, 1-20.

Berke, D. (1991). *Network Structure, Support Functions, and Satisfaction with Social Support: An Analysis of the Convoy Model for Individuals and Families.* Unpublished Ph.D. Dissertation. University of Delaware.

Beutler, I., & Burr, W. (1989). A seventh group has visited the elephant. *Journal of Marriage and the Family, 51*, 826-829.

Bienstock, C., & Videka, S. (1989). Process analysis of a therapeutic support group for single parent mothers: Implications for practice. *Social Work with Groups, 12*, 43-61.

Blieszner, R. (1988). Individual development and intimate relationships in middle and late adulthood. In R. Milardo (Ed.), *Families and social networks* (pp. 147-167). Beverly Hills, CA: Sage Publications.

Bond, C., & Daiter, S. (1979). Participation in medical self-help groups. In M. Lieberman, & L. Borman (Eds.), *Self-help groups for coping with crisis* (pp. 164-180). San Francisco: Jossey-Bass.

Borman, L. (1982). Self-help skills: Leadership in self-help mutual aid groups. *Citizen Participation, 3*, 30-31.

Boss, P. (1993). The reconstruction of family life with Alzheimer's disease: Generating theory to lower family stress from ambiguous loss. In P. G. Boss, W. J.

Doherty, R. LaRossa, W. R. Schumm, & S. K. Steinmetz (Eds.), *Sourcebook of family theories and methods* (pp. 163-166). New York: Plenum.

Burant, R. (1989). The "families" focus of Families in Society. *Social Casework, 70,* 523-524.

Call, D. (1990). School-based groups: A valuable support for children of cancer patients. *Journal of Psychosocial Oncology, 8,* 97-118.

Caplan, G. (1976). The family as support system. In G. Caplan, & M. Killilea (Eds.), *Support systems and mutual help: Multidisciplinary explorations* (pp. 19-36). New York: Grune & Stratton.

Caplan, G., & Killilea, M. (1976). *Support systems and mutual help: Multidisciplinary explorations.* New York: Grune & Stratton.

Chesler, M., Barbarin, O., & Lebo-Stein, J. (1984). Patterns of participation in a self-help group for parents of children with cancer. *Journal of Psychosocial Oncology, 2,* 41-63.

Chilman, C., Cox, F., & Nunnally, E. (Eds.). (1988). *Employment and economic problems, families in trouble series (Vol. 1).* Newbury Park, CA: Sage Publications.

Cobb, S. (1976). Social support as moderator of life stress. *Psychosomatic Medicine, 38,* 300-314.

De Araujo, G., Van Arsdel Jr., P., Holmes, T., & Dudley, D. (1973). Life change, coping ability, and chronic intrinsic asthma. *Journal of Psychosomatic Research, 17,* 359-373.

Dean, A., & Lin, N. (1977). The stress buffering role of social support. *Journal of Nervous and Mental Disease, 165,* 403-417.

Durman, E. (1976). Role of self-help in service provision. *Journal of Applied Behavioral Science, 12,* 433-444.

Edwards, G., Hensman, C., Hawker, F., & Williamson, V. (1966). Who goes to Alcoholics Anonymous? *Lancet, 2,* 382-384.

Enright, A., Butterfield, P., & Berkowitz, B. (1985). Self-help and support groups in the management of eating disorders. In D. Garner, & P. Garfinkel (Eds.), *Handbook of psychotherapy for anorexia nervosa and bulimia* (pp. 491-512). New York: Guilford.

Footlick, R. (1989, April 22). Redefining the family. *New York Times,* p. 18Y.

Fried, B. (1976). Alcoholics Anonymous as a self-help group: Institutionalized but not professionalized. Unpublished manuscript, University of Chicago.

Froland, C., Pancoast, D., Chapman, N., & Kimboko, P. (1981). *Helping networks and human services.* Beverly Hills, CA: Sage Publications.

Gartner, A., & Reissman, F. (1977). *Self-help in the human services.* San Francisco: Jossey-Bass.

George, L. (1987). Non-familial Support for Older Persons: Who is Out There and How Can They Be Reached? In G. Lesnoff-Caravaglia (Ed.), *Handbook of applied gerontology* (pp. 310-322). New York: Human Sciences Press, Inc.

Gibeau, J. (1986). *Breadwinners and caregivers: Working patterns of women working full-time and caring for dependent elderly family members.* Unpublished Ph.D. dissertation. Brandeis University.

Gonyea, J. (1989). Alzheimer's disease support groups: An analysis of their structure, format and perceived benefits. *Social Work in Health Care, 14*, 61-72.

Greene, D., McVinney, L., & Adams, S. (1993). Strengths in transition: Professionally facilitated HIV support groups and the development of client symptomatology. *Social Work with Groups, 16*, 41-54.

Hartley, P. (1988). The role of self-help groups in eating disorders. In D. Scott (Ed.), *Anorexia and bulimia nervosa: Practical approaches* (pp. 177-191). Washington Square, NY: New York University Press.

Hinrichsen, G., Revenson, T., & Shinn, M. (1985). Does self-help work? An empirical investigation of scoliosis peer support groups. *Journal of Social Issues, 41*, 65-87.

Holstein, J. A., & Gubrium, J. (1999). What is family? Futher thoughts on a social constructionist approach. *Marriage & Family Review*, this volume.

Johnson, C. (1988). Relationships among family members and friends in later life. In R. Milardo (Ed.), *Families and social networks* (pp. 168-189). Beverly Hills, CA: Sage Publications, Inc.

Katz, A. (1970). Self-help organizations and volunteer participation in social welfare. *Social Work, 15*, 51-60.

Katz, A. (1981). Self-help and mutual aid: An emerging social movement? *Annual Review of Sociology, 7*, 129-155.

Katz, A., & Bender, E. (1976). *The strength in us: Self-help groups in the modern world*. New York: New Viewpoints.

Knight, B., Wollert, R., Levy, L., Frame, C., & Padgett, C. (1980). Self-help groups: The members' perspectives. *American Journal of Community Psychology, 8*, 53-65.

Koroloff, N., & Friesen, B. (1991). Support groups for parents of children with emotional disorders: A comparison of members and non-members. *Community Mental Health Journal, 27*, 265-279.

Krauss, M., Upshur, C., Shonkoff, J., & Hauser, P. (1993). The impact of parent groups on mothers of infants with disabilities. *Journal of Early Intervention, 17*, 8-20.

Leach, C. (1990). ALS support groups: An update. *Loss, Grief and Care, 4*, 201-225.

Leveton, L., Griffin, R., & Douglas, T. (1979). Social supports and well-being in urban elderly. Unpublished manuscript.

Levy, L. (1976). Self-help groups: Types and psychological processes. *Journal of Applied Behavioral Science, 12*, 310-322.

Levy, L. (1982). Mutual support groups in Britain. *Social Science in Medicine, 16*, 1265-1275.

Levy, L., & Derby, J. (1992). Bereavement support groups: Who joins; who does not; and why. *American Journal of Community Psychology, 20*, 649-662.

Lieberman, M., & Borman, L. (1979). *Self-help groups for coping with crisis: Origins, members, processes, and impact*. San Francisco: Jossey-Bass.

Lowenthal, M., & Haven, C. (1968). Interaction and adaptation: Intimacy as a critical variable. *American Sociological Review, 33*, 20-30.

Marcenko, M., & Smith, L. (1991). Post-adoption needs of families adopting children with developmental disabilities. *Children and Youth Services Review, 13,* 413-424.

Maton, K. (1994). Moving beyond the individual level of analysis in mutual-help group research: An ecological paradigm. In T. Powell (Ed.), *Understanding the self-help organization* (pp. 136-153). London: Sage Publications.

McAfee, W. (1952). *Alcoholics Anonymous: An evaluative study.* Unpublished doctoral dissertation, University of Chicago.

Milardo, R. (Ed.). (1988). *Families and social networks.* Beverly Hills, CA: Sage Publications, Inc.

Nuckols, K., Cassel, J., & Kaplan, B. (1972). Psychosocial assets, life crisis, and the prognosis of pregnancy. *American Journal of Epidemiology, 95,* 431-441.

Ramey, J. (1988). Intimate vs. non-intimate support networks. In S. Steinmetz (Ed.) *Family and support systems across the lifespan.* New York: Plenum Press.

Ramsey, P. (1992). Characteristics, processes, and effectiveness of community support groups: A review of the literature. *Community Health 15* (3), 38-48.

Rubel, J. (1984). The function of self-help groups in recovery from anorexia nervosa and bulimia. *Psychiatric Clinics of North America, 7,* 381-394.

Settles, B. H. (1987). A perspective on tomorrow's families. In M. Sussman and S. Steinmetz (Eds.), *Handbook of marriage and the family* (p. 157-180). New York: Plenum Press.

Shumaker, S. & Brownell, A. (1984). Toward a theory of social support: Closing conceptual gaps. *Journal of Social Issues, 40,* 11-36.

Smith, K., Gabard, D., Dale, D., & Drucker, A. (1994). Parental opinions about attending parent support groups. *Children's Health Care, 23,* 127-136.

Telleen, S., Herzog, A., & Kilbane, T. (1989). Impact of a family support program on mothers' social support and parenting stress. *American Journal of Orthopsychiatry, 59,* 410-419.

Toseland, R., & Rossiter, C. (1989). Group interventions to support family caregivers: A review and analysis. *The Gerontologist, 29,* 438-448.

Vaux, A., & Athanassopulou, M. (1987). Social support appraisals and network resources. *Journal of Community Psychology, 15,* 537-556.

Videka-Sherman, K. (1982). Effects of participation in a self-help group for bereaved parents: Compassionate friends. *Prevention in Health Services, 1,* 69-77.

Weiss, R. (1973). *Loneliness: The experience of emotional and social isolation.* MA: MIT Press.

Wheat, P., & Lieber, L. (1979). *Hope for the children.* Minneapolis, MN: Winston.

Williams, T. (1985). *Family life events, perceived stress, and social support utilized: An examination of sex differences.* Unpublished Ph.D. Dissertation. Michigan State University.

Zimmerman, S. (1988). *Understanding family policy: Theoretical approaches.* Newbury Park, CA: Sage Publications.

The Process of Family Therapy: Defining Family as a Collaborative Enterprise

Anthony Jurich
Lee N. Johnson

INTRODUCTION

The time is 5:55 p.m. on a winter's evening at the Family Therapy Clinic at Kansas State University. Tony and Lee have looked over the "pink intake sheet," compiled from the initial telephone interview with the family, and have conversed about the nature of the case. The entire process pertaining to the case, however, has been held in abeyance until the arrival of the family for their first therapy session. Until the family arrives for therapy and begins to define, not only the nature of the problem but also the nature of the family, all other speculations, formulations, and strategies for intervention must be suspended. This process of defining the family by family members during therapy is unique in each case. People involved may include family members who are present and absent, people from their psychosocial environment, and one or more "helping service agencies." Unlike research or theory in which the theoretician or researcher holds the decision-making capability for defining "family," during therapy this process is shared by family members and the therapist. Whether done overtly through specific discussion or covertly by inclusion or omission, the process of defining the family has a major impact on the therapy that this family has sought. It is a cornerstone upon which the

Anthony Jurich and Lee N. Johnson are affiliated with the Kansas State University Department of Human Development & Family Studies, Justin Hall, Manhattan, KS 66506.

[Haworth co-indexing entry note]: "The Process of Family Therapy: Defining Family as a Collaborative Enterprise." Jurich, Anthony, and Lee N. Johnson. Co-published simultaneously in *Marriage & Family Review* (The Haworth Press, Inc.) Vol. 28, No. 3/4, 1999, pp. 191-208; and: *Concepts and Definitions of Family for the 21st Century* (ed: Barbara H. Settles et al.) The Haworth Press, Inc., 1999, pp. 191-208. Single or multiple copies of this article are available for a fee from The Haworth Document Delivery Service [1-800-342-9678, 9:00 a.m. - 5:00 p.m. (EST). E-mail address: getinfo@haworthpressinc.com].

191

rest of therapy will be built. It is 6:00 p.m., and the clients are arriving–so let the process begin.

Systems Theory

The starting place for most family therapists in defining "family" would be Systems Theory, a perspective that, at its base, conceptualizes families' interactional systems. Watzlawick, Beavin, and Jackson, for example, have put forth the following: "An interactional system was defined . . . [as] two or more communicants in the process of, or at the level of, defining the nature of their relationship" (1967, p. 153). This approach defines family at its most elemental level. Members of the family system are refining the definition of their family relationships in an ongoing process through the interactive use of communication. System theory breaks the family down to its most basic components, without which the family system would not exist. However, it does not tell the reader some very important information, such as:

1. Who is included within the family system;
2. How are family members related to one another;
3. What kinds of communication are utilized;
4. Do these communications form patterns that are recognizable; and
5. Who is responsible for the family system's equilibrium?

We propose that these questions are determined for every specific family by the particular family members involved. Moreover, when the family enters therapy, the therapist also makes a contribution. Both the family and the therapist bring to the sessions a set of expectations, based upon previous experiences, training, and presumptions, from those who form their psychosocial environment. We will attempt to elaborate some of the salient factors both the family and the therapist bring to the process of definition.

THE FAMILY

Each family brings to the definitional process an input from each family member, their collective group experience as a family, and their interpretation of society's expectations. Even fairly objective definitions, such as those based on biological or legal criteria (Schwartz, 1993), must be filtered through the psychosocial filter of the family's experience, both individually and as a unit. A woman who is raped may give birth to a child and, therefore, be biologically and legally linked to that child as the mother but may have a very different psychosocial interpretation of that child as a member of her family. To further complicate the matter, the psychosocial interpretations of a legal or biological event may be quite different among family members. In the example of the raped woman, she may embrace the child within her definition of family, only to have her husband reject the child as "somebody else's bastard." From a sociological point of view, this is obviously a view of family rooted deeply within symbolic interaction (Stryker, 1964). Because the individuality of each family is of paramount importance to the therapeutic process, however, a symbolic interaction framework is deemed to be not only appropriate but necessary.

Next we will address how the family brings its preconceived notions of the definition of family to the therapeutic process. Within this discussion, we will try to address the five questions posed above that reach beyond the basic definition from Systems Theory.

Who Is Included Within the Family System?

For most families, the starting place for the definition of whom is included in the family is, "All the members of a household; those who share one's domestic home" (Morris, 1969: 474). Some families may have very rigid boundaries and may exclude any people not living within the domestic home, even if they may be legally or biologically linked to the family. These might include aging parents in nursing homes or children away at college. The rigidity of the boundaries may "cut off" a potential family member and exclude him or her from the self-defined family (Kerr, 1981). Likewise, a family may also have very rigid and inclusive boundaries. These families may include adult children who have long since grown and moved out on their own or close next-door neighbors within their definition of "family," even though they may have no legal or even blood ties to the family. These families are "enmeshed" with these self-defined members and describe themselves as being "incomplete without them" (Kerr, 1981). In either case, the rigidity of the boundary is paramount, and the family enters into the therapy sessions with an inflexible, preconceived definition of their family. This creates a "closed system" that often tries to ". . . prevent new information, new options, and new resources from entering and challenging the family system" (Harber, 1987:269).

Other families may have much more permeable boundaries that let the definition of who is in the family be much more flexible (Minuchin, 1974). A college student may be considered to be "launched" when he or she is away at school but again part of the family when he or she returns home for the summer. However, a family may have a boundary that is so diffuse that family membership appears to be a moment-to-moment event. One day, the parents of the child's best friend may be considered part of the family, because the children spend *so* much time together. The next day, the child might be expelled from the family for uttering a four-letter word.

Between the "rigid" and "diffuse" boundary families lie the majority of families. The boundaries of these families are flexible but have enough rigidity to help define who is inside the family and who is not. Because many of the families who seek family therapy are having difficulties in coping with their lives, the family therapist may see more families at the extremes of the continuum. Either their extreme boundary style has caused them difficulties for which they are seeking therapy or a family problem has caused them to become more extreme in their style of boundaries as either a defense or coping technique. In either case, the family therapist is more likely to be faced with a family for whom boundary maintenance is a problem.

Laying aside the relative rigidity of family boundaries, there are a number of other factors that may determine whether an individual is placed within or outside of the boundaries that divide the family. Age may become a determining factor of who is included in the family. Because of the importance of peers to the adolescent (Jurich, 1987), the adolescent may define his or her best friend as a member of the family, regardless of other family members' acceptance of the idea. Older people, especially those whose families have passed away, often define significant people in their lives, such as friends or caretakers, as being "family" (Genevay, 1992). Often families from different cultural backgrounds will include extended family members as central to their definition of "family." This has been found to be true of families in Japan (Okado, 1990) and Kenya (Wilson, 1982). In our own culture, this tendency to include the extended family has been found among Mexican-American (Soto, Sylvia, & Robert, 1994) and Navajo (Topper & Curtis, 1987) families. Such inclusions of extended family members or friends may be very important to one or more family members in the definition of the family who is coming in for therapy. This is further complicated by the fact that not all family members may agree upon whether to include or exclude a given individual. This will further escalate the tension within the family.

Forces outside the family's control may have an effect upon who is defined to be within the family. A family may want their delinquent son to be part of their family and to attend therapy sessions. However, the son's actions have gotten him into trouble with the law and he is not available because of his incarceration. The family may agree with this incarceration and appreciate that a disruptive force in the family is no longer present. Another possibility is that the family may feel badly that their son is no longer with them, but validate the legal authorities' right to incarcerate their son. They may also feel as if the authorities "were too hard on him" and defiantly keep him within the family "in spirit." A painful vacuum may be created in a family by a grandmother who lived with them for years, but then suddenly was taken to the hospital or a nursing home.

The ultimate in "forces outside the family" is the death of a family member. The family may have a difficult time not including their deceased loved one in the family. In extreme cases, the family may launch into denial and keep the family member alive within the family. The family could resort to the use of symbols to keep the family member alive. For example, the senior author had a case in which the family would not let anyone sit in the dead family member's favorite chair in an effort to keep a sense of the deceased family member's presence still in the house. How the family reacts to these externally-caused inclusions or exclusions is very important to their self-definition. Are they accepting of the situation; do they challenge or fight it; or do they deny it even took place?

Finally, there are idiosyncratic situations that give rise to inclusions or exclusions within the family's definition of "family." A certain series of events may lead a family to include or exclude individuals from the family situation. For example, having a child launched into a new family of their own through marriage may tug at some heartstrings, but can basically be a joyful graduation of the youth from the family. The lover of one of the spouses, however, may intrude into the family with an extremely unwanted presence. A stepsister may join the family to the joy of all in the family, except for one stepbrother.

Family members may be jettisoned because of infractions of family rules. After performing some valued task, such as getting a job, a family "black sheep" may be reintegrated into the fold. Father may be left at home, while mom and the children are forced to flee to a shelter because of his abuse. Mother may be considered to be a part of the family only if she is not inebriated. Pets may be considered to be little more than "breathing furniture" or may hold a place in the house on a par with the humans. Even inanimate objects, such as the television, may be considered to be a valued baby-sitter or a barbaric invader of the sanctity of the home. Because these situations *are* so idiosyncratic, the therapist has to be aware that each family's definition of self is both unique and valued by the family as a definition of reality. Whether stated overtly or covertly, the family will have some very definite ideas as to who resides within the boundaries of the family system.

How Are Family Members Related to One Another?

In the previous section, much of the text referred to the family as if it were one person. The authors tried to point out that although there were times when the family members did indeed act with one accord, there are also times when there is disagreement among family members or between factions of family members. Although the symptomatology of the family or of any single family member will affect *every* family member, each will be affected to a different degree and, at times, in different directions (Bodin, 1981). Consequently, part of the family's self-definition is not only who is included within the family but how they relate to each other.

Families often see themselves as subdivided into smaller groupings within the family (Minuchin, 1974). These family sub-systems are formed in an effort to maintain the homeostasis that the family defines as a "steady balance" within the larger family system (Guttman, 1991). If a father was to be authoritarian, his wife and children may feel fairly powerless to bring about their own wishes within the family system. Consequently, the wife and children could form a sub-system coalition in an effort to equalize the power in reference to the authoritarian parent. Consequently, the family defines itself as a series of separate but connected sub-systems (Minuchin & Fishman, 1981).

Typical sub-systems within a family are the parental or executive sub-system and the sibling sub-system (Minuchin, 1974). In a typical family, the adults (the parents) in the system cooperate together to lead the family and make decisions that will be beneficial to the entire family. To counterbalance that sub-system, the children may form a sibling sub-system to give each other support and comfort in the face of the typically more powerful parental sub-system. Many families seeking therapy do not possess such a typical balance of sub-systems and some do not have an executive sub-system. Despite the fact that there may be one or two parents present, no adult leadership is taken and the family steers rudderless through life. In other families, one or more children may ascend into an executive sub-system, because the parents refuse to assume control of the family. Still other families may form a coalition between an adult and a child to create an executive sub-system. Following a divorce, for example, such circumstances may occur for adolescents and custodial parents who must assume leadership of new single-parent families (Jurich & Jones, 1986). In dual-parent families, such advancements of children into the executive sub-system often occur with the corresponding fall of one of the parents into the sibling sub-system. Consequently, sub-systems within the family may determine the hierarchy within the family and the relative power held by each family member.

Power within the family may not, however, be distributed in a "top-down" manner, but also might be wielded from a "one-down position." The overt power of the executive sub-system, for example, coincides with the overt responsibility for the rest of the family system. Consequently, a person in a "one-down position" within the family can often force family members in the executive sub-system to yield to his or her wishes by broadcasting his or her own vulnerability and by asking (really demanding) that the executive sub-system take care of his or her needs. Instead of a game of "one-upmanship" in which each participant tries to "top" the other, a game of "one-downmanship" is created in which case each participant tries to be more wounded so that the other is forced to take care of him or her. Thus, the use of family sub-systems not only defines what the relationships among the family members are but also determines the flow of power in the family.

What Kinds of Communication Are Utilized?

"Knowledge and meanings are the product of interactions between persons" (Anderson & Goolishian, 1991, p. 22) and these interactions express themselves through communication. Family members cannot "not communicate" (Watzlawick et al., 1967), with communication taking on several different forms.

Most often when one thinks of communication within families, one thinks of the dialogues that take place between and among family members. Most often one pays attention to the literal meaning of the words that are spoken, the lexical content of the speech (Jurich & Polson, 1985). This language allows family members to make sense of their experiences and organize them (Anderson & Goolishian, 1991). These experiences are put together through stories and narratives. In this way, descriptions and interpretations are created, refined, and modified as the family defines and redefines itself through its own dialogue. In this way, meaning is given to the family experience and the family is continually defined.

A given family may have several stories or narratives that express the nature of strong and heroic women within the family. That theme will now become part of the definition of the family. A family in therapy typically has coalesced around some problem within the family. Consequently, the family has created a problem-organizing language system that it utilizes to define itself. A family with an alcoholic father will begin to define themselves as "broken" and tell stories that exemplify the problem of dad's drinking and the family's inability to cope with the alcoholism. These narratives may be born out of some new crisis or may dovetail with previous family narratives, some of which may have been passed down through the generations.

Suppose we combine the two examples we have put forth in the previous paragraph. A family that has several narratives about strong and heroic women finds itself tossed into crisis by an alcoholic father. We would expect that this family's self-definition through its narratives would prompt one or more of the family's women to come forth and try to help the family cope with the alcohol-induced crisis. In some cases, this may aid the situation and prompt the family to create a new narrative. In most of the families who are seen in family therapy, there would be minimal relief from the "problem" and even the old adaptive narratives might support a problem-solving language system.

In addition to the lexical content of the speech, family communication has nonlexical and nonverbal components to the communication (Jurich & Polson, 1985). These components of communication make up the "metamessage" of the communication or the "message about the message" (Watzlawick et al., 1967). They explain to the listener how he or she is to take the message conveyed by the lexical component of the communication. A cheerful message said with a smile and a carefree tone of voice gives the listener a congruent message to understand. However, a cheerful message spoken with sarcasm and venom is confusing, because the listener does not know whether to believe the message that is cheerful or the metamessage that is not. The message said by a family member who is seeking to manipulate another family member by playing "martyr" may appear to be benign, because it is encouraging the listener to do something for himself or herself. However, the martyr will include a metamessage that induces guilt if the more benign message of the lexical text is followed. Consequently, the listener is double-bound, because the messages seem to contradict each other. In most cases, the listener will pay attention to the more powerful metamessage and will acquiesce to the speaker's wishes. However, the listener will also feel resentful or very confused by the interchange and feel worse about the interpersonal relationship. Families entering therapy often have confusing messages, contradictory messages, and metamessages that poison their communication and, hence, their definition of the family.

Do These Communications Form Patterns That Are Recognizable?

The communications in which the family members engage do not occur at a single place in time. Moreover, narratives are responded to by other family members. Feedback is given to the narrator so that the story may be altered and refined (Watzlawick et al., 1967). The narrator then responds to the listener's feedback, and the listener gives more feedback to that response. In this way, communication within the family settles into a recursive cycle that may or may not be recognized by the family as occurring (Haley, 1987).

Many families entering therapy have established "maladaptive recursive cycles," or patterns that do not work and have become dysfunctional for one or more family members. Many families entering therapy define their families by the types and frequencies of these maladaptive recursive cycles. Often they do not fully understand the nature of these cycles, but each family member knows when one is beginning and demonstrates this knowledge by increased anxiety at the expectation of another poor outcome. This, of course, adds to the feelings of crisis and the definition of the family as being problematic, unable to function, and broken.

Who Is Responsible for the Family System's Equilibrium?

"A family is organized to maintain the organization that defines it as a family" (Keeney, 1983: 86). The family will seek to ensure the survival of the family as they have defined it. Consequently, most family members will desperately try to hold onto the family as they know it and have defined it. They will maintain the family system's homeostasis so that they may continue to operate within a set of rules that determine the range of behavior that may vary within the family (Guttman, 1991). Consequently, on one level, the family believes that they have the locus of control over the equilibrium of the family *within* the family. Family members believe that they control their own destiny. However, the family members also assume that they can control their own destiny by minimizing the amount of disruptive influence upon the family. They do this by promoting the homeostasis or the *status quo* of the family.

This would be a viable option if it were not for the fact that families are not "closed systems" that tend toward homeostasis. Instead, families are "open systems" that tend to progress toward morphogenesis, the state of growing and elaborating (Buckley, 1967). Open systems, like families, change because they take in new energy and information from the outside. Moreover, open systems, like families, change because they grow. Children grow up; people age and die; and the system is forced to change, with change being the only constant in this type of system. Some families are aware or become aware of this press towards morphogenesis, but most families assume that homeostasis *can* be achieved and *should* be pursued. In most families, when things are going well, homeostasis seems achievable, and the family feels that they have the power and responsibility for the family system's equilibrium. However, when things start to go badly and the family's narratives become problem oriented, it becomes easy to see how these family members would feel out of control. Some no longer feel as if they had the power and, consequently, the responsibility for the change within the family system. Most families come into family therapy believing that they are relatively helpless and that the power of change lies not within the family or its members, but outside the family and, most likely, with the family therapist. A key element, therefore, is that therapy is frightening, and the therapist is an intimidating presence within the family.

THE THERAPIST

The therapists must initially be reactive to the situation presented by the client. Consequently, the therapist must wait to see the situation presented by the client's family before any therapeutic formulations or speculations can be advanced. This includes the client family's definition of itself. However, even before the family steps foot into the room, the therapist will have some preconceived ideas as to how he or she will define a family who enters into therapy. These preconceptions often have their origins from two main sources: (a) the school of therapy to which the therapist adheres, and (b) the personal therapeutic style of the therapist.

Schools of Family Therapy

There are many schools of family therapy, but all of them have an underlying allegiance to the principles of Systems Theory. As stated at the beginning of this paper, a family is an interactive, open system, whose members are perpetually defining themselves by means of their communication (Watzlawick et al., 1967). Some basic systemic rules are prevalent, such as the whole system is greater than the sum of its parts (Buckley, 1967) or "nowhere among living organisms can one find 'unattachment'" (Minuchin & Fishman, 1981:14). However, each school of Family Therapy subscribes to a theory that emphasizes certain aspects of the "family" definition over other aspects that might be deemed important by a different theory.

Behavioral Family Therapy. Behavioral Family Therapy emphasizes the behavioral omponents of the family's communication (Falloon, 1991). What family members say about their family is not nearly as important as how they act. Behavioral patterns are analyzed as to the preconditions to the behavior, the behavior itself, and the succeeding rewards or punishments the system gives to that behavior. Contingency contracts are established and monitored for their effectiveness in changing the problem behavior. This contract is drawn up under the guidance and supervision of the therapist, but the responsibility for implementing the change rests with the family members involved. How family members are related to one another is not an important issue for the behavioral family therapist. Instead, the inclusion or exclusion of any given family member is only important in so far as that individual has the ability to establish preconditions or contingently reinforce the problem behavior. Except for the ability of the therapist to help direct the establishment of the contingency contracts or to reinforce certain behaviors with social approval, the therapist is not seen as a major part of the family system.

Intergenerational Family Therapy. Intergenerational Family Therapy has its roots in Psychoanalytic Theory and draws upon the client family's individual members and their relationships with family members in their families of origin (Kerr, 1981). The intergenerational aspects of the family are considered to be of paramount importance. Even when the presenting problem is confined to a single generation, such as a marital problem, the focus will still reach out to the extended family of the family of origin for both spouses (Framo, 1981) and to the children presently in the home (Boszormenyi-Nagy & Ulrich, 1981).

Some proponents of these types of intergenerational therapies actually expect the family to bring these extended family members into therapy (Framo, 1981). Others believe that family therapy can be accomplished without the physical presence of those extended family members in the sessions but that the client's family must focus on those intergenerational interactions and may be given homework assignments to confront those extended family members between therapy sessions (Kerr, 1981). In either case, it is obvious that the inclusion of the extended family, especially from the client family's families of origin, is a key part of the Intergenerational therapist's definition of the family.

The way that all of these extended family members are related to each other and their patterns of communication are focused upon in the therapy sessions (Kerr, 1981). The therapist is interested in symbiotic role patterns, such as the overfunctioner-underfunctioner role-pair, and in coalitions that form triangulation patterns in which the communication between two family members is channeled through a third family member in order to reduce anxiety. For the most part, Intergenerational therapists focus on the lexical portion of the communication with the clients. The intergenerational therapist's role is to analyze and educate the client family and the therapist may set up an occasional homework assignment. Despite this active role, the responsibility for change is centered around the individual family members and their determination to change patterns of family interaction learned from families of origin.

Structural Family Therapy. Structural Family Therapy focuses on the change in family structure, as opposed to individual change being the main goal of therapy (Minuchin, 1974). The structural family therapist studies the patterns of interactive communication in order to understand the underlying structure and organization of the family system. Consequently, the kinds and patterns of communication are important only for determining how the family members are related to one another structurally. Issues of sub-systems (spousal, parental, and sibling), coalitions, and hierarchies are of paramount importance in both understanding family problems and in giving direction to changing families.

Structural family therapists also study boundaries within the family to determine whether they are rigid, clear, or diffuse. The therapist brings about change in the system by studying the family's structure and assigning a series of tasks to the family that are designed to loosen some of the sub-system's boundaries, while tightening other boundaries (Minuchin & Fishman, 1981). In this manner, sub-systems are altered and refined into a pattern that is more suitable to less problematic family functioning. The therapist has the primary responsibility for both change and equilibrium within the family. In this way, the family will establish an executive hierarchy and be able to better cope with family problems.

Strategic Family Therapy. Strategic Family Therapy focuses on the clinical family's maladaptive recursive cycles that manifest themselves in the communication patterns of the family members' interactions (Haley, 1987). Strategic family therapists advocate seeing the entire family so that all these recursive communication patterns can be observed and analyzed. Any family member who contributes to the maladaptive pattern, whether they are nuclear or extended family, is defined as part of the family for the purposes of doing therapy, and they may be asked to participate in the therapeutic sessions. In some cases, the strategic family therapist might even venture beyond the legal or blood lines of the family and include people close to the family patterns of communication, such as adolescent peers (Selekman, 1991).

Strategic Family Therapy is also very concerned with the types of communication utilized, although it is less interested in the specific sub-systems among family members except for how they contribute to communication patterns. Because it is assumed that the family members will try to maintain the homeostasis of the family system (Guttman, 1991), the strategic family therapist expects that the family will try to resist any change to the present system, regardless of how dysfunctional that system's patterns of interaction may be. Consequently, the therapist has the responsibility to ". . . design the most appropriate and effective therapeutic intervention" (Watzlawick & Weakland, 1977: xiv). Subsequently, the Strategic Family Therapist has the obligation to take action to implement that intervention in such a way as to overcome the family's homeostatic inertia and set a course for therapeutic growth (Fisch, Weakland & Segal, 1982). Consequently, the therapist becomes an integral part of the family system and has the responsibility of being the prime mover for change.

Constructivist Family Therapy. Constructivist Family Therapy focuses on the family's continuing redefinition of itself and assumes that the family system includes the therapist as a new "player" in the system who is also attempting to redefine the family on a continuing basis (Keeney, 1983). In fact, with the advent of Health Maintenance Organizations and Managed Care Systems, the Constructivist Family Therapist would argue that the family definition in therapy must now include another level of supervisors and bureaucrats who currently join in defining the family system in a way never before experienced (Friedman, 1989). The Constructivists are most interested in stories and narratives about the family as the basis for a mutual search for understanding that is conducted by the family and the therapist (Anderson & Goolishian, 1991). The focus is on the lexical component of communication and the meanings that families attach to these narratives rather than on any specific patterns of communication or structures or sub-systems. The mutual exploration of the family's stories leads to " . . . new meaning, new narrative, and new agency" (Anderson & Goolishian, 1991, p. 23). The therapist's responsibility is to create a space in which the therapeutic conversation can occur and be facilitated. The responsibility for change, however, is a shared process.

Obviously, the school of family therapy to which the therapist subscribes will have an enormous impact on the way the family is defined in the therapeutic process. To complicate matters further, very few family therapists adhere religiously to only one school of family therapy, with most having two or more styles from which they draw. This further complicates the definition of a family within the therapeutic process.

Therapist's Personal Style. Over and above the specific school or schools of family therapy that a therapist follows, each therapist has an idiosyncratic style that may have major implications for the "family's definition." Some therapists are much more comfortable working with only one or two people in the room. Others feel at home with a large number of people in the therapy session. Obviously, the latter therapist will be much more comfortable with a family with fairly diffuse boundaries and may encourage a family to define its membership well beyond the nuclear family. The former therapist may not only restrict the family's definition of family, but also restrict who is in the room for therapy, pushing for individual family member sessions instead of seeing the whole family.

Some therapists are very reluctant to assume any responsibility for the family's equilibrium. They prefer to be respectful of the client family's right to decide the nature, speed, and direction of the change process. Other therapists feel that it is their duty to take primary responsibility to bring about change in the family system. Some therapists are very efficient in their therapy and push the family to change quickly, while others are much more patient, preferring to let the client family change at its own pace. These idiosyncratic styles of the family therapists further complicate the definitional process in therapy.

THE THERAPY PROCESS

Obviously, there are at least two sets of preconceived expectations that enter into the room at the time of the first therapy session. Regardless of the therapist's school of family therapy or personal style, the first attempt at defining a family in therapy belongs to the family. Before the therapist is even seen, it is the family who decides who will arrive for therapy, how they will present their problem, and who will be assigned responsibility for the problem. It is the therapist who must wait for the family's "opening move" and convey respect to the client family for their formulation of the problem by trying to understand the problem as the client family sees it. The family, by the act of entering therapy, has taken a courageous journey to a foreign land, the world of therapy and professional helpers. They are indeed strangers in a strange land. Furthermore, because the expectation is that they will open up and express their innermost thoughts and feelings to the therapist, this journey into therapy is a journey with very high stakes. They have a lot to gain–a more satisfying family life–but they also have a lot to lose, revealing vulnerabilities to a stranger or, even worse, to themselves.

The power of intimidation that is associated with the first therapy session is provided when the problem of male clients (husbands or fathers) entering therapy is considered. Many professionals have decried the dearth of adult males coming into family therapy. We search for answers by indicating that, even today, women have the primary responsibility for the maintenance of caretaking functions within families (Losh-Hesselbart, 1987). Consequently, it is argued that more women come into therapy, because the therapist is expected to help them with their typical family role. However, another set of dynamics appear to be at work on adult male family members that are relevant to the family's definition of itself. Traditionally, males have held the protective role in families (Nye & Berardo, 1973), with part of this task being concerned with boundary maintenance. Although much of the protective function within families has been given over to outside agents (police and military services), the remnants of that tradition still linger on in families of today. Consequently, the adult male in families (husband, father) still carries the functional obligation to maintain the family boundary.

Adult females (wives, mothers) are allowed, on the one hand, to seek therapy for assisting with the task of expressive leadership within families. In contrast, the very act of seeking therapy often is used to "prove" the male adult's inability to do his assigned job of boundary maintenance, because the boundary has been violated by an invader–the therapist. Consequently, the very act of participating in therapy is an admission of the husband/father's failure to protect the boundary of the family. Consequently, many men would rather not participate in therapy, which, by definition, is an admission that they have failed by allowing the therapist to invade the family boundary and be defined as a family member.

Once the family communicates the initial definition of their family, the therapist must validate this definition and work both overtly and covertly with the family during therapy so that expansion can occur and elements of his or her own family definition can be included. The family's presenting complaint may be one of discipline problems with the child. After a session or two, the therapist may begin to believe that the family's problem has little to do with children or discipline, but instead is a marital problem in which the husband and wife are engaged in a power struggle. As correct as the therapist's view may be, the family will seldom abandon their view of the situation and automatically accept the therapist's definition. This family must be invited to consider the therapist's definition of the family and be told that they have the option to reject that view. Although a discordant definition of the family and its presenting problem may initially be rejected, some information has been passed on to the family simply by mere suggestion. New information has been added to the system, with an important result being that homeostasis has been challenged. If the therapist continues to believe that this family is indeed suffering from a marital problem, he or she can reinvite the family to consider a different definition of their family. Even if they reject the therapist's definition a second, third, or even fourth time, the very act of challenging the family's definition begins to change the definition of the family and mold it into a more shared vision of the family.

There may be times when a family member whom the family therapist believes to be essential for inclusion as a family member cannot or will not come to therapy. The family therapist must decide if he or she will acquiesce to the family's definition and exclude the person. Another possibility is to push the family to change their definition and accept the therapist's point of view. A third alternative consists of reaching a compromise, such as by setting up an "empty chair" for the missing family member so a presence can be maintained, even though they are physically absent from the family.

Circumstances in the therapeutic process may mandate that the family therapist engineer a change in the family definition. The therapist may ask the family to expand its definition of family to include the friend of an adolescent who may be able to help move the family therapy process along (Haber, 1987; Selekman, 1991). Such a suggestion may need to undergo negotiations as the family tries to feel comfortable with this change in their self-definition. The request for inclusion of a non-family member to be admitted into the family in therapy may also come from a family member. An aging family member may ask the therapist to include a dear life-long friend in therapy in an effort to create a family since the biological family may no longer be available (Genevay, 1992). In this case, the therapist must display sufficient flexibility to alter his or her own definition of the family to accommodate the family member's request. In still other circumstances, the request for a change in family definition is made by medical or legal emergencies. An adolescent whom the courts send to a hospital for treatment is taken out of the family definition, at least physically. However, the family must now include the hospital staff and therapists as new members of its expanded family definition, even though neither the family therapist nor the family itself sought to change that definition (Withersty, Porterfield & Spradlin, 1975). Such an integration of the hospital staff and therapists into the family's self-definition aids in the family's sharing responsibility and working cooperatively with the hospital.

Negotiating the definition of the family in therapy is of crucial importance in today's world in which the traditional two-parent nuclear family is dwindling as the norm (Schwartz, 1993). Single-parent families and blended families make the process of defining family even more complicated and often volatile. A single-parent family may want to specifically exclude a non-custodial parent who has visitation rights and is still a major influence on the child. A blended family may want to forget the non-custodial biological parents whose different house rules keep the children in a constant state of disruption after visitations. An unwed father may be excluded from all therapy by the unwed mother's parents. In each of these situations, the family therapist may view it in the best interest of the client family or a specific member of the client family to expand the boundaries of the family for the sake of therapeutic change. This negotiation with the family may be quite logical or it may be extremely emotional. In either case, it will be slow and the therapist will have to be both respectful and patient. However, even if the family does agree to alter its working definition of the family, it is also important, for legal purposes, to remain clear as to the therapist's definition of who is the client. Simply because a family agrees to expand its family definition to include an ex-spouse for the sake of therapy, does not mean that that ex-spouse is now also the therapist's client. These distinctions must be made clear to all concerned, because the legal obligations to the original client family must take precedence over the expanded therapeutic family if the therapist is called to court. The fact that collaboration in family therapy is set within a legal framework is not a minor concern.

This is obviously a very complicated and idiosyncratic process of defining the family in a therapeutic process. The therapist must take into account the family's previous definition, their expectations, and his or her own preconceptions that are based in a particular school of family therapy and personal style preferences. Once these parameters are set, the therapist and family must embark on an ongoing negotiation process of definition and redefinition. The ultimate goal is that the therapist will learn from the client family about how they define themselves as a family. Subsequently, the therapist must apply skill and training to assist the family to redefine itself and bring about therapeutic change. A therapeutic perspective is used to reflect back to the family a more pleasing and satisfying mirrored image of themselves than that which they began with at the onset of therapy.

REFERENCES

Anderson, H., & Goolishian, H. (1991). Thinking about multi-agency work with substance abusers and their families: A language systems approach. *Journal of Strategic and Systemic Therapies, 10* (1), 20-35.

Bodin, A. M. (1981). The interactional view: Family therapy approaches of the Mental Research Institute. In A. S. Gurman & D. P. Kniskern (Eds.), *Handbook of family therapy: Vol. 1* (pp. 267-309). NY: Brunner/Mazel.

Boszormenyi-Nagy, I., & Ulrich, D. N. (1981). Contextual family therapy. In A. S. Gurman & D. P. Kniskern (Eds.), *Handbook of family therapy: Vol. 1* (pp. 159-186). NY: Brunner/Mazel.

Buckley, W. (1967). *Sociology and Modern Systems Theory.* Englewood Cliffs, NJ: Prentice-Hall.

Falloon, I. R. H. (1991). Behavioral family therapy. In A. S. Gurman & D. P. Kniskern (Eds.), *Handbook of family therapy: Vol. 2* (pp. 65-95). NY: Brunner/Mazel.

Fisch, R., Weakland, J. H., & Segal, L. (1982). *The tactics of change: Doing therapy briefly.* San Francisco, CA: Jossey-Bass Publishers.

Framo, J. L. (1981). Marital therapy with sessions with family of origin. In A. S. Gurman & D. P. Kniskern (Eds.), *Handbook of family therapy: Vol. 1* (pp. 133-158). NY: Brunner/Mazel.

Friedman, S. (1989). Brief systemic psychotherapy in a health maintenance organization (HMO). *Family Therapy, 16* (2), 133-144.

Genevay, B. (1992). "Creating" families: Older people alone. *Generations, 16* (3), 61-64.

Guttman, H. A. (1991). Systems theory, cybernetics, and epistemology. In A. S. Gurman & D. P. Kniskern (Eds.), *Handbook of family therapy: Vol. 2* (pp. 41-62). NY: Brunner/Mazel.

Haber, R. (1987). Friends in family therapy: Use of a neglected resource. *Family Process, 26,* 269-281.

Haley, J. (1987). *Problem-Solving Therapy (2nd Ed.).* San Francisco, CA: Jossey-Bass Publishers.

Jurich, A. P. (1987). Adolescents and family dynamics. In H. G. Lingren, L. Kimmons, P. Lee, G. Rowe, L. Rottmann, L. Schuab & R. Williams (Eds.), *Building family strengths: Vol. 8.* Lincoln, NE: University of Nebraska Press.

Jurich, A. P., & Jones, W. C. (1986). The worst of times to be: The effects of divorce upon adolescence. In J. Leigh G. & Peterson (Eds.), *Adolescents and Families.* Cincinnati, OH: South-Western.

Jurich, A. P., & Polson, C. J. (1985). The nonverbal assessment of anxiety as a function of level of intimacy of sexual attitude questions. *Psychological Reports, 57,* 1247-1253.

Keeney, B. P. (1983). *Aesthetics of change.* NY: Guilford Press.

Kerr, M. E. (1981). Family systems theory and therapy. In A. S. Gurman & D. P. Kniskern (Eds.), *Handbook of Family Therapy: Vol. 1* (pp. 226-264). NY: Brunner/Mazel.

Losh-Hesselbart, S. (1987). Development of gender rules. In M. B. Sussman & S. K. Steinmetz (Eds.), *Handbook of Marriage and the Family* (pp. 535-563). NY: Plenum.

Minuchin, S. (1974). *Families and family therapy.* Cambridge, MA: Harvard University Press.

Minuchin, S., & Fishman, H. C. (1981). *Family therapy techniques.* Cambridge, MA: Harvard University Press.

Morris, W. (Ed.). (1969). *The American heritage dictionary of the English language.* Boston, MA: American Heritage Publishing Company and Houghton Mifflin.

Nye, F. I., & Berardo, F. M. (1973). *The family: Its structure and interaction.* NY: MacMillan.

Okado, T. (1990). Perspectives on family psychology in Japan: First international symposium of family psychology. *Japanese Journal of Family Psychology, 4* (special issue), 39-53.

Schwartz, L. L. (1993). What is a family? A contemporary view. *Contemporary Family Therapy, 15* (6), 429-442.

Selekman, M. (1991). "With a little help from my friend": The use of peers in the family therapy of adolescent substance abusers. *Family Dynamics of Addiction Quarterly, 1* (1), 69-76.

Soto, F., Sylvia, D., & Robert, L. (1994). Structural family therapy with Mexican-American family systems. *Contemporary Family Therapy and International Journal, 16* (5), 349-362.

Stryker, S. (1964). The interactional and situational approaches. In H. T. Christensen (Ed.), *Handbook of Marriage and the Family* (pp. 125-170). Chicago, IL: Rand McNally.

Topper, M. D., & Curtis, J. (1987). Extended family therapy: A clinical approach to the treatment of synergistic dual anomic depression among Navajo agency-town adolescents. *Journal of Community Psychology, 15* (3), 334-348.

Watzlawick, P., & Weakland, J. (1977). *The interactional view: Studies at the Mental Research Institute, Palo Alto, 1965-1974.* NY: W. W. Norton & Company.

Watzlawick, P., Beavin, J. H., & Jackson, D. D. (1967). *Pragmatics of human communication.* NY: W. W. Norton & Company.

Wilson, N. R. (1982). Family therapy in Kenya. *Journal of Family Therapy, 4* (2), 165-176.

Withersty, D. J., Porterfield, P. B., & Spradlin, W. W. (1975). Treating the hospitalized adolescent: A family approach. *Family Therapy, 2* (2), 129-135.

Definitions of the Family:
Professional and Personal Issues

Barbara H. Settles

INTRODUCTION

In the field of family studies, many useful definitions of the family have been developed to meet the scholarly, professional, and policy needs of the past (Settles, 1987). Usually textbooks have begun with a review of such definitions and the authors often pick the definition they will support in their analysis of families. In research, the reports often specify how families were identified for the study or whether a stand-in for family such as household or house address was used. While it has been argued that households are functionally equivalent to families for the purposes of governmental data, this assumption is difficult to test as the data are not delineated to do this task. Many of our research reports on family are limited to family as seen by one member of the family or at most the perception of a dyad or two within the group. If there ever was a consensus on the definition of the family, it is not to be found in today's research and policy analysis. Whether the operational definitions, which have served us well for specific projects, should be or could be integrated or abstracted to produce a clear conceptual definition for the field at a theoretical level is under debate. *The political and social consequences of conceptualizations of family are potent.*

In family studies there has been a concern for communicating our findings from research and applying theory and research to family problems and family challenges in an accurate and appropriate way. This has led us to be aware of the theoretical and methodological difficulties in defining family

Barbara H. Settles is affiliated with the Department of Individual and Family Studies, University of Delaware, Newark, DE 19716.

[Haworth co-indexing entry note]: "Definitions of the Family: Professional and Personal Issues." Settles, Barbara H. Co-published simultaneously in *Marriage & Family Review* (The Haworth Press, Inc.) Vol. 28, No. 3/4, 1999, pp. 209-224; and: *Concepts and Definitions of Family for the 21st Century* (ed: Barbara H. Settles et al.) The Haworth Press, Inc., 1999, pp. 209-224. Single or multiple copies of this article are available for a fee from The Haworth Document Delivery Service [1-800-342-9678, 9:00 a.m. - 5:00 p.m. (EST). E-mail address: getinfo@haworthpressinc.com].

209

both in the research and the applications. What family? When? For what purpose? All are recurrent problems. Two early incidents in my own work drew my attention to the substance of the family conceptually and as an issue in reality: (a) my dissertation and (b) my first paid consultancy.

PERSONAL AWARENESS
OF DEFINITIONAL ISSUES IN FAMILIES

In my dissertation (Settles, 1964), which was a part of a much larger study on younger families with children, I conducted intensive interviews with families who had younger children. I had been assigned the rural fringe target population, those who had chosen to build homes in the metropolitan area, not in conventional suburbs, but often a corner or the frontage of a farm. One of the objectives of the larger project was to examine how communities influenced the family life and so the protocol emphasized community participation and informal contact. When I began my study, the general questionnaire included questions about three friends most frequently visited.

Rogers (1995), in his pioneering work on successful farmers in the highly technical large scale farms in Iowa, developed a theory of how innovations spread. He noted the visiting patterns of those who were early adopters of new ideas and found that both their contact with academic and friendship networks were widespread from their farms and that both their technical and life style choices were drawn from far-flung networks. In Ohio, where I was completing my doctorate work at Ohio State University, policy makers in the state legislature were concerned about urbanization and the relationships of new families in rural areas to the communities.

I began doing the long and complex interviews in the homes and reviewed the protocols. When I was coding the data, I realized that something was not quite right. I did a few callbacks and from the discussion developed another question for probe: *How many of these friends are also family?* In the majority of these rural families the overlap was that most, if not all, close friends were also family related. This indicator was then useful in looking at the concepts of familism and visiting patterns as some of the more tested and conventional scales in the protocol for predicting other family behaviors. At a Groves Conference on Marriage and the Family, in her plenary address, Hareven (1991) noted that the overlap between the concepts of friends and family is a long-standing one historically and that our current desire to keep these ideas completely separate is not supported by data from even recent past. Therefore, the usual assumptions about these concepts of family and friends being truly separate entities was not and is currently not sustainable.

The second incident occurred when I was asked to the evaluation of a War on Poverty program demonstration of a self-governed youth service center in the inner city of Columbus, Ohio (Settles, 1967). Of course, this program was a highly political one that had come into being because an African-American church had taken the initiative to apply for funds to support a program that they were already committed to developing. When we (the research team) began to conduct a study of the membership as promised in the proposal, we attempted to contact the young people at the addresses that they had given on their membership cards. The interviewers were faced with the way teenagers actually lived in this community. The comments included:

- No, he's not here, he stayed over at his aunt's.
- Oh, she's living over at her boyfriend's now.
- Don't know where he is this week.
- No, they moved.
- I think his mom put him out. Check over at the Laundromat.
- They had a fight and he left.
- Her uncle was after her f_____[sexually] so she ran away.

Even before homelessness was rediscovered in the eighties, poor families did not often find it easy to maintain households and teenagers had especially high "vapor points" for leaving their families early and often. This concept of household as family, so often used in census and demographic studies, has always had some slippage and appears to be even more problematic for the future.

Defining the family as a concept for the future requires not only a re-examination of the traditional understanding of family, but also of what is involved in defining a concept. When Betty Friedan (1963) suggested that she had found a problem for which there was no name, that is, the "feminine mystique," the framing of this concept became the proving ground for the debate of a new feminist movement. Jesse Bernard (1983) reports a similar experience in the response to her work on academic women (1964). By the second edition of her book many readers and reviewers had pointed out to her that she had laid out a field of study by her analyses so others could work to develop it. The need to have a vision for the spaces in between the current ideas is a challenge to the theoretician. The spaces among the conceptions of family and families need to be addressed.

PROFESSIONAL CHALLENGES IN DEFINING THE FAMILY

Education for family studies and professional practice is found in a number of disciplines, professional schools, and interdisciplinary programs. In the current climate of academic restructuring finding the name and descriptions of offerings that provide appropriate experiences and academic preparation is a challenge. Certainly, as a field the study of "family" is rapidly growing, and opportunities for work and leadership are plentiful. Because this field has many strands of development, even professionals are frequently not fully aware of how the different groups have handled similar issues and concerns. In family studies, the ongoing work of defining and redefining the family has had both broad political and narrow substantive impact. In the greater society debates about family policy and programs reflect ideological cleavages in the body politic. Family research and programs may enter these discussions, but usually as an illustration for an already structured position.

In the academy, family scholars may be surprised to discover how controversial their work may be to the audiences to whom their administrators must be accountable. In each country and region of the world these greater and lesser controversies over family as ideology and reality are played out in different ways. Sometimes it is by what is not done: lack of funding, choice of samples, limited questions, limited discussion of topics, elimination or consolidation of programs or positions. Sometimes it is by what is rewarded: prestige and recognition in one's career, availability of human and material resources, protected speech and inquiry, freedom and support to travel and publish. While we recognize that those places we characterize as totalitarian states may limit both the academic inquiry and the public discussion of family concepts and values, clearly everywhere, family is a topic of importance in values and assumptions about the good society. There are many unintended and often unforeseen outcomes to each finding we disseminate about families, and our theoretical interpretation may have consequences in the larger political arena as well as in our standards of best practice.

While American academic life has its own provincialism, it does influence the scholarly processes elsewhere. Family studies does exist openly in the university system as well as other levels of the school system. It is frequently a primary career identification although it is also a secondary or interdisciplinary identification to many other scholars. In any university there may be several groups that have some enterprises in family studies and the players may or may not know each other or interact. It is quite common to meet a colleague at a national or international professional meeting and exclaim that you have not seen them since last year although you are at the same institution. Therefore the illustrations given here may be of interest in the United States as well. To learn from the conflicts and challenges of some of these separate programs may be helpful in illuminating why family definitions are such politically and emotionally riveting concerns. Some professional examples will be given from family science, family therapy, family history, family sociology, nursing, and interdisciplinary family studies to illustrate the critical necessity for being alert to the consequences of family concepts in shaping opportunities and limitations families encounter. Family definitions serve many purposes in the various family-centered professions. Research, practice and educational applications make different demands on theory for specificity, universality and sensitivity to practical issues.

THE WAY FAMILY IS DEFINED:
ETHICAL CODES AND BEST PRACTICE

Family therapy, as a profession, is now facing the issues around defining family and especially how therapeutic outcomes should be evaluated. Although the first marriage counseling centers were established in the thirties and professional standards emerged in the fifties, recent growth has led to expansion and consolidation of training and accreditation of professionals as therapists. Different intervention strategies have grown up side by side that have diverse ideas about success. Minuchin, for example, freely adapted from sociology the Parsonian structural-functional ideas about the standard nuclear family and set forth some strong recommendations about families maintaining boundaries between generations and characterizing stability and behavioral change as an appropriate outcome (Kaslow, 1987). Kaslow also notes that Bowen, on the other hand, drew attention to the extended kinship network and focused on resolving multigenerational issues as the focus for both the treatment and evaluation of outcome.

The focus of professional efforts has not been to build consensus on a definition or model. Rather more emphasis has been given to development of ethical codes and policies which create respect for family diversity and some peace among practitioners with divergent techniques and objectives (Hardy & Nickles, 1987; Kaslow, 1987). Another source of pragmatism among family therapists has been the need to keep order among the group to promote standards for third party payments and professional recognition (Leigh, Lowen & Lester, 1989). Therapists have studied the individual, active families who present themselves for assistance. The return of case studies and individual family analysis has been at the forefront of publication in the therapy journals and now is also finding its way, as qualitative methodology, back into the sociology and general family studies journals. Jurich and Johnson (see their article in this volume), discuss how therapeutic intervention and familial definitions are negotiated in therapeutic practice.

The need for ethical codes and consensus about best practice is not limited to therapists. Family life educators, social workers and sociologists have also developed codes and certifications to deal with the increased efficacy of their intervention strategies and the public expectation that quality is not only possible, but can be demonstrated. Among the points made in these codes and certifications is that families deserve the best knowledge and skills we have and that their integrity and life choices deserve respect.

THE WAY FAMILY IS DEFINED:
BENCHMARKS, LIFE COURSE AND MACRO-LEVEL ANALYSIS

Family history emerged in the 1960s as history scholars began to reconstruct life patterns of ordinary people. Family history has blossomed and scholars have tried to link the micro level individual data to large-scale demographic analysis. For example, such scholars as Hareven, Elder, Ullenberg, and Hogan have influenced interdisciplinary and international work in the family by calling attention to the misreading of the past and the likelihood of misunderstanding current data when one approaches it with inaccurate assumptions about the past base line information, and the life course of individuals and their families (Hareven, 1996). Elder (1981) notes that complexity is enhanced by greater historic analysis. Coontz (1992) analyzed the recent past of the '50s families and brushed away many of the assumptions about the nuclear family of that period. An increased awareness of individuals and families having histories themselves that include different cultural periods and social change has affected our view of the family. For example, many of the working moms of the '60s and '70s were also the stay-at-home moms of the '50s. As Jesse Bernard (1983) pointed out in examining the female world in global perspective, women have many more recurrent choices and years in which to enact changes. Family historians have suggested more caution in attributing changes in family life to technological or social events and examined families as also a source of change and active agents in their contacts with the forces of change (Hareven, 1987).

Family sociology, traditionally, has had a pragmatic view of family. It had been appropriate to take whichever standard definition one admired, as well as a definition which could be adapted to the research or intervention at hand. One could refer to it and use for the study, making any adjustments necessary depending on what household data was available. Large numbers of cases were thought to be valuable to wash out any minor variations. The essence of hypothesis testing was in trends and similarities, not in differences and diversity. The wide variety of studies and techniques used reflects this practical bent.

The search for commonalties in social systems for macro-theoretical presentations in sociology created an enterprise of collating and codifying across cultural and historical periods the structure and functions of families. Lee (1987) draws our attention to Murdock's 1949 concept of the nuclear family as providing four functions, regulation of sexual relations, reproduction, primary socialization and economic cooperation between husband and wife, which he considered to be universal. The universality of the nuclear family, however, has been questioned by more recent analysis. Lee (1987) maintains that nuclear family systems as opposed to the overall frequency of nuclear families everywhere are not so likely in low-technology agriculturally based societies, but occur frequently at both the simplest hunting/gathering levels and most complex high technology societies, a curvilinear function. Burgess's definition of a "unity of interacting personalities" dominated the output of studies on the family according to Mogey (1981, in Thomas & Wilcox 1987:84). Sociological pragmatism stemmed from a concern about social problems and the role of a "fragile family" in handling the impact of larger social forces (Thomas & Wilcox, 1987).

Osmond (1987: 119-122) in her review of radical-critical theories suggested that the understanding of the politics of theory building itself could be helpful in opening up a less static view of family. She believed that gender has not been taken seriously and that examining families "as processes that contain the interplay of contradictory forces, which can result in disorganization and radical change," would be important and would encompass the variety of existing families.

Complex statistical analyses are interesting at the macro-level of policy choices; however, they are only as useful as the choice of theory that orders the analysis. Sociologists' interest in macro explanations of social stability and change created a driving force that made it easy to propose overly simple family definitions of nuclear and extended families. In this schema social support networks were all that was necessary to capture the qualities of family and friends in contemporary society.

The politics of a gender revolution and methodological shift that refocuses attention on the dyadic and small group expressions of cultural forces has affected many family studies areas in addition to sociology. Both the swift growth of life course oriented areas such as childhood and aging and the sweep of gender studies and diversity are challenging the usual measures of quality and importance in the field. At the same time a new wave of traditional thought and practice has dominated the political life and activities of the profession of sociology. Etzioni's (1993) advocacy of communitarian response to modern alienation and breaks in the social support of individuals and families became the agenda of the American Sociological Association's annual meeting in 1995 when he was president.

Currently many conservative leaders idealize a traditional nuclear family, but protest characterizing this stand as antifeminist. Whether or not these opinion leaders will counter the most recent wave of feminist change and historic research is still unsettled. At this moment in time family sociology cannot stand on the grounds of non-political objective science as its strategy.

Family is at the center of politics today. Survival of family sociology is dependent on a pro-active approach.

THE WAY FAMILY IS DEFINED:
CENSORSHIP AND CURRICULUM

Family and Consumer Science, as it is now called, derives from home economics, and was one of the first professional disciplines to grapple with issues of values in understanding families. Historically, the field had a professional concern bordering on an obsession with having a consensus on what was meant by family and a familial centered program for home economics (Brown, 1985). The national association spent considerable energy and money bringing together their leaders to redefine both the concepts of family and of the discipline at several points in the twentieth century. The Lake Placid Conferences (1899-1908), which are usually seen as the founding of the field, left a heritage of concern for the family even as its implementation was sometimes a narrow view of rational homemaking (Brown, 1985). Ellen Richards' (also know as Ellen Swallow-Richards) poetic description of family in home economics remained important to the profession throughout its development (Parker, 1983).

Home Economics:

- ideal home life for today unhampered by the traditions of the past.
- utilization of all resources of modern science to improve the home life.
- freedom of the home from the dominance of things and their due subordination to ideals.
- simplicity in material surroundings which will most free the spirit
- for the more important and permanent interests of the home and of society. (Ellen H. Richards–1904 [Founder & First President AHEA])

This concern was in these concepts: (1) Home economics works through the family to effect an optimum balance between people and their environments. (2) Home economics accepts the challenge of helping people adjust to change and to shape the future (American Home Economics, 1959). Brown (1985) believes that naiveté prevented the profession from addressing the critical issues especially those related to individual and family life because the problems of families were shallowly conceived. East (1980:165) said simply, "A family is a group of people who care about each other," and then went on to a list of "usuallys," which gathered up a wide variety of other definitions to arrive at the conclusion that home and family are complex and reverse concepts somewhat independent of each other. She concluded (1980:174), "After all people live together in families because of love not logic." In the following decade the association reorganized itself to highlight this concern for serving families and renamed itself the American Association of Family and Consumer Sciences. In recent years the issue of what it means to serve families and to build that effort on informed research and policy analysis remains a challenge.

While this family scientist approach to definition is far too broad to be useful in specific research or theorizing, it has served the professional association (AAFCS) well in keeping a broad scope of service and programs to a wide variety of households and familial groups. What was at risk in this debate and consensus building was the political necessity for family and consumer sciences as a professional field not to be captured or limited as a group to promoting a single family form or helping politicians determine who is eligible for programs by eliminating groups that were not conventional or "traditional nuclear families."

This was especially important for their role in public school secondary education. In American schools, three types of books are particularly open to criticism and outright censorship: biology, government, and family and consumer sciences textbooks (del Fattore, 1992; Holden, 1987; Nelkin, 1976). Family and consumer science textbooks have been criticized for their humanistic content. Censorship has been particularly aimed at those texts that deal with family and the processes in the family and individual related to decision making and values. For teachers, definition of family has not been a side issue but one of surviving as a profession against political pressures and limitations. Currently, they face the problem of having specific and inclusive understandings of family in developing national standards for accountability in consumer and family programs in middle and secondary schools (Liprie, 1998).

Secondary level teaching is often limited in its freedom to discuss controversial topics in other fields, not just family and consumer sciences. It is important to look at family studies offerings in higher education in general. This issue is now being engaged in college level texts that cut across interdisciplinary family studies. Glenn (1997a) has taken up the "neo-liberal," "communitarian" or perhaps really neo-traditional cause in critiquing family texts for the Council on Families in America. His approach was two-fold, attacking texts on (a) "scholarly" grounds of balance, accuracy of presenting contrasting views, and arguments from evidence and (b) attention to the treatment of selected issues of the importance of marriage, effects of families, especially solo parents on children, and analysis of the debates on family change and feminism. While this kind of presentation looks like a research and book review exercise, it is primarily a political tract to set the grounds for new guidelines in publication for the collegiate level. Censorship is often not necessary if the atmosphere is chilled before a text writer begins to write.

As Skolnick (1997) notes in her rejoinder to Glenn, at the center of the culture wars is the issue of defining the family, who is to be included and excluded from our world view and moral visions. One of the problems of those who have more tolerant comprehension of families is that they cannot believe they should be arguing over conserving social patterns that are not either what they were idealized as or prevalent in the ways posited by neo-traditionalists. Therefore the field of debate is usually defined by the advocates of a narrow view of family and family structure and function. Being in a reactive mode makes it easy for one to be drawn into the others' schema. As is usual in debate format Glenn (1997b) has a second chance to address his rejoinders and can slip away from their arguments to protest he has no agenda to shape the texts. When it comes to citation indexes and media coverage, the ability of advocates for narrow family definitions to be quoted and to be paid attention to their approach is quite startling. (Note that by discussing this issue, I have increased their citation index count!)

There are many other examples from family science about controversial family values and definitional quandaries such as sexuality education, decision making and planning, abuse prevention and intervention, gender and cultural diversity programming. In each of these areas the political and community context subject the individual professional to risk, controversy and professional threat.

THE WAY FAMILY IS DEFINED:
TECHNICAL, LEGAL AND MORAL STRAINS

Among the groups who have recently adopted an expanded interest in family studies have been the founding members of the university life: medicine, law, and philosophy. Technical advancements in all areas of life have changed the opportunities, risks and decision making processes for individuals and families. Whether attention should be paid only to individuals or primarily to families or some moderate stance is an increased problem as change moves along. Whether and how the community or nation-state enters into this arena is also controversial.

One example that includes all three aspects is rapidly changing health and well-being aspects of medical intervention. Traditionally in western medicine the emphasis in treatment had become the individual within a medical institution. The relationship between the type of technology and the role of the individual and family in medical treatment and decision making has become more complex. The movement in medicine toward professionalization and expert based institutional care that characterized health care in the earlier years of the twentieth century has been challenged by both a declining confidence in institutions and a need to address the dynamic process of care and cost over the life course (Pescosolido & Kronenfeld, 1995).

Transitions back and forth between the formal care system and informal care are mediated by a number of social processes and perceptions and information sources (Haug, 1990). The completion of a huge number of tuberculosis hospitals after World War II was followed almost immediately by their desertion due to successful medical treatment on an out-patient basis. Now the system is faced with helping out-patients who do not have a family support network cope with out-patient treatment in order to stem the growth of resistant tuberculosis. The disinstitutionalization of the mentally ill also demonstrated the shift in how medical intervention is to be delivered.

The return of the patient to the home at much earlier stages of treatment with a substantial demand on the family for more than just companionship and social support has become established practice, with even greater possibilities predicted for the near future (Dolan, Caeynne, & Simpson, 1989). A patient who has no close friends and/or family who will provide care may be in grave difficulty. Coombes (1991) reviews the literature on marital status and posits a protective hypothesis to explain why single status is associated with major physical and psychological health problems.

The care situation, the caregivers' reactions, and their outcomes in emotional health all influence the continuance of care (Ellis, Miller & Given, 1989). In treatment for cancer and AIDS, questions about suppressed immune systems have been answered by suggesting that home care is safer during the treatment, but that immediate, speedy, and appropriate hospitalization is critical when indicated. The role of the family and friends in assessment as well as care requires sophisticated patient and caregiver education. The breadth of demands on family, by the new technologies and choices is immense in its diversity, power, and difficulty. Legal issues arise around such topics as informed consent, providing consent for those who are not able to give consent, dealing with conflicts of interest and privacy. Moral issues are found when cost and benefits are estimated, treatments are managed or rationed, when individual, family, and community perspectives are weighed.

Medical alternatives for individuals and families increasingly erase the boundary between home and institution and the course of medical treatment and prevention over the life course has made the family into the case manager for the individual. Advocacy, support and direct caregiving are now major roles that individuals must develop intimate networks to handle. Those without concerned and active families are at risk in the current medical alternatives. Defining family as it interacts with health, well-being, and medical institutions continues to be highly controversial. For example, currently intensive care units in hospitals limit visiting to the intimate family and usually simply ask that first on the scene to list the family. This list then functions as a social contract and usually works well enough except for those with diverse family forms or conflict-ridden family relationships. However, if the same process was used for financial responsibility, there might well be legal action and signatures not so easily secured. The fact that these medical-health questions require knowledge and skills not available through tradition challenges the style and substance of ordinary family norms and decision-making processes.

THE WAY FAMILY IS DEFINED: INTERDISCIPLINARY STUDY AND COLLABORATION

Throughout academic and governmental institutions the trend has been to encourage interdisciplinary family study and practice. Team provision of services and programs has been found to be an efficient model in family services. Because of the wide variation of family definitions and conceptualizations in the various branches of family scholarship these interdisciplinary projects are often fraught with conflict. If scholars or practitioners trained in different theories and methods do not work through conflicts, they quickly descend to calling each other incompetent and fail to get the synergy desired in bringing together different expertise. When interdisciplinary projects include an objective of being international or cross-cultural in their application, finding the words to express meaning not simply to translate language is a major concern. While family may be found everywhere today, the use of terms like pro-family and pro-choice illustrate how important words are in the political dialogue. To use family nomenclature to describe relationship in complex organizations like churches and voluntary associations is another indicator of the power of the imagery of the family. Advertisers of products and promoters of causes and programs both use the wealth of meanings of symbols like the family to attach some of these meanings to the acceptance of these products and ideas.

"Family" is a term that one first incorporates into one's vocabulary as a young child and it appears early on spelling lists in the primary grades. We cannot strip a word or idea of these early layers of meaning without being presumptuous. It is likely that we are doomed to failure to communicate a new understanding of families outside our modest group of scholars unless we deal with these prior meanings. Ownership of terms and their use is a constant political struggle both inside the discipline and in the larger political arena.

Creating a definition of family studies has provided a case study in bringing scholars together. Burr and Leigh (1983) with their colleagues attempted in the early eighties to define family scholarship in terms of a discipline and proposed a name, familogy, based on the approach so many areas of study have used to create a technical name for the fields. Burr argued that the body of information, theory, and practice had become substantive enough and similar training was being used broadly for those who saw themselves as family scholars. His proposal received a lot of response and some of it was quite negative. However in the shake out, many activities and projects emerged from these debates about discipline, a section was organized in the National Council on Family Relations to address the discipline, the American Home Economics Association was renamed American Association of Family and Consumer Sciences, and the Family Science Association was founded and will have its 11th anniversary meeting this year. Apparently, family science evolved as the term that best captured this vision of family studies and scholarship. Integration of concepts and uses of family as an independent entity with characteristics of process and outcomes specific to itself seems to have dominated the movement.

PERSONAL AND PROFESSIONAL COMMITMENTS TO THE OPEN DIALOGUE IN SCHOLARSHIP IN FAMILIES

There are disadvantages to clarity and reliability in defining a concept that is of value to many audiences. The exclusionary process of clarifying may limit the utility of the concept to users. Stretching ideas and words to fit new situations is a familiar strategy in developing new ideas. In the academic marketplace there are many forces that might constrain the dialogue and necessary discussion of families and processes of defining and developing concepts about families. No field has as many reasons to attend to the nurturing of academic freedom and faculty involvement in governance of the university. Free speech and tolerance are fundamental to our work. Inclusion and diversity in the professoriate and the student body are basic to inclusion and diversity in family studies. It has been recognized that part of the responsibility of individual scholars and their organizations is to assure that these principles are honored at every level of the scholarly enterprise. Now it is also clear that the consequences and interpretation of research findings and theory in the political market place should cause us to become more involved in the public policy uses of our work. While one cannot take every controversy or application, some responsibilities accrue to the "housekeeping" needed to keep an open and inclusive academic and public conversation.

The current highly charged discussion of family definitions in the public sphere has had many precedents in family studies. As a professional, my first real encounter with the power of political and social movements was in the repression of family life sexuality education at the end of the sixties. When in 1969 a committee of our Delaware State legislature wrote to me demanding my graduate course syllabus, list of movies and other teaching materials, and texts for a series of community hearings, I realized that in-service education for teachers was a super-hot topic and that any comparative or non-value laden framework was suspected of undercutting the social good. I was protected to some extent by my institution's aversion to being a totally state institution and my provost wrote a pleasantly strong letter saying no to the request, but suggesting they drop in anytime they wanted to visit my class. I taught that summer under the threat of immediate publicity and possible professional injury. This encounter was only the beginning of taking responsibility for the freedom to speak and teach. Over my career in family studies in an institution of higher education, I have found myself needing to be a local political activist for a number of issues related to my freedom to be a scholar in family studies.

Human sexuality in my institution was treated as an interdisciplinary teaching effort by a group of scholars who developed a course in the early '70s. It ran successfully for 17 years, until in another budgeting change, we had to find a home for it to be funded, and brought it into the Individual and Family Studies Department. Now in 1998, I am once more on a committee to examine whether we will be allowed to teach human sexuality in this department. Does sexuality have anything to do with individuals and families? Does a definition of family speak to human sexuality? The challenge in this area never is over. Women's studies, ethnicity and diversity issues, and international programs are other areas in which it has been important that academic freedom and opportunity be preserved for family studies to flourish.

Faculty governance and representation are at the foundation of any academic freedom, scholars have to pursue topics, such as family definition, that have political consequences. Only in a free and open academic setting can we examine families as an abstraction, a reality and as an advocacy issue. Professional challenges to the way the family is defined include:

- Developing professional ethical codes and refining best practice.
- Identifying families as they change across the life course and in historical perspective.
- Resisting censorship and limitations to family studies curriculum.
- Helping families and institutions cope with the technical, legal, and moral issues of a rapidly changing milieu for family decision making.
- Finding an intellectual and equitable basis for interdisciplinary family studies.

At the personal level scholars need to attend not only to their own research and programs, but also to the academic and societal level to ensure a foundation for open discussions.

REFERENCES

American Home Economics Association (1959). *New Directions.* Dorothy D. Scott (Committee chair). Washington, DC: AHEA.

Bernard, J. (1983). *The development of Women's Studies and Family Sociology: An Interview with Jessie Bernard: With B. H. Settles and M. L. Liprie* [Videotape]. (Available from University of Delaware, Newark, DE 19716).

Bernard, J. (1964). *Academic women*. University Park: Pennsylvania State University Press.

Burr, W. R., & Leigh, G. T. (1983). Familogy: A new discipline. *Journal of Marriage and Family, 45*, 467-480.

Brown, M. M. (1985). *Philosophical studies in the United States* (Vols. I & II). East Lansing, Michigan; Michigan State University.

Coombes, R. H. (1991). Marital status and personal well-being: A literature review. *Family Relations 40*(1), 97-102.

Coontz, S. (1992). *The way we never were: American families and the nostalgia trap*. NY: Basic Books.

del Fattore, J. (1992). *What Johnny shouldn't read: Censorship in America*. New Haven, CT: Yale University press.

Dolan, B., Caeynne, S. C., & Simpson, J. E. (1989, July 31). Sick and tired. *Time*, pp. 48-53.

East, M. (1980). *Home Economics, past, present, and future*. Boston: Allyn and Bacon.

Elder, G. H. (1981). History and the family: The discovery of complexity. *Journal of Marriage and Family, 43*, 489-520.

Ellis, B. H., Miller, K. I., & Given (1989). Caregivers in home health care situations: Measurement and relations among critical concepts. *Health Communication, 1*(4), 207-226.

Etzioni, A. (1993). *The spirit of community: The reinvention of American society*. NY: Simon and Schuster.

Etzioni, A. (1996). The responsive community: A communitarian perspective. *American Sociological Review, 61*(1), 1-11.

Friedan, B. (1963). *The Feminine Mystique*. NY: Macmillan.

Glenn, N. D. (1997a). A critique of twenty family and marriage and the family textbooks. *Family Relations, 46*(3), 197-208.

Glenn, N. D. (1997b). A reply to Cherlin, Scanzoni and Skolnick; Further discussion of balance, accuracy, fairness, coverage, and bias in family textbooks. *Family Relations, 46*(3), 223-226.

Hardy, K., & Nickles, W. (1987). *Ethical Codes in the Family*. Paper presented at the N.C.F.R. Meeting. Detroit, MI.

Hareven, T. (1987). Historical analysis of the family. In M. B. Sussman & S. K. Steinmetz (Eds.), *Handbook on marriage and the family*. NY: Plenum.

Hareven, T. (1991). *Friendship, family and kin in historical perspective*. Paper presented at the Groves Conference on Marriage and the Family. Panama City, FL.

Hareven, T. (Ed.) (1996). *Aging and generational relations over the life course: A historical and cross-cultural perspective*. Berlin: Walter de Gruyter.

Haug, M. R. (1990). The interplay of formal and informal health care: Theoretical issues and research needs. *Advances in Medical Sociology, 1*, 207-231.

Holden, C. (1987, January 2). Textbook controversy intensifies nationwide. *Science, 235*, pp. 19-21.

Holman, T. B. (1980). Beyond the beyond: The growth of family theories in the 1970's. *Journal of Marriage and the Family, 42*, 729-741.

Kaslow, F. W. (1987). Marital and family therapy. In M. B. Sussman & S. K. Steinmetz (Eds.), *Handbook on marriage and the family.* NY: Plenum.

Lee, G. A. (1987). Comparative Perspectives. In M. B. Sussman & S. K. Steinmetz (Eds.), *Handbook on marriage and the family* (pp. 59-80). NY: Plenum.

Leigh, G., Lowen, I. R., & Lester, M. E. (1986). Caveat Emplori: Values and ethics in family life education and enrichment. *Family Relations, 35*(10), 573-580.

Liprie, M. L. (1998, May). Personal communication on her participation in the National Standards Commission of Family and Consumer Sciences.

Nelkin, P. (1976, April). The science textbook controversies. *Scientific American, 234*, pp. 33-40.

Osmond, M. W. (1987). Radical-critical theories. In M. B. Sussman & S. K. Steinmetz (Eds.), *Handbook on marriage and the family* (pp. 103-124). NY: Plenum.

Parker, F. J. (1983). *Home Economics: An Introduction to a dynamic profession* (2nd ed.). NY: Macmillan.

Pescosolido, B. A., & Kronenfeld, J. J. (1995). Health, illness, and healing in an uncertain era: Challenges from and for medical sociology. *Health and Social Behavior* (extra issue), 5-33.

Rogers, E. M. (1995). *Diffusion of innovations* (4th. ed.). NY: The Free Press.

Skolnick, A. (1997). A reply to Glenn: The battle of the textbooks–Bringing in the cultural war. *Family Relations, 46*(3), 219-222.

Settles, B. H. (1964). *Factors affecting the familial orientation of young families in a rapidly urbanizing area of Franklin County, Ohio.* Unpublished doctoral dissertation. The Ohio State University, Columbus, OH.

Settles, B. H. (1967). *Youth civic center final report.* USHEW unpublished.

Settles, B. H. (1987). A Perspective on tomorrow's families. In M. B. Sussman & S. K. Steinmetz (Eds.), *Handbook on marriage and the family* (pp. 157-180). NY: Plenum.

Thomas, D. L., & Wilcox, J. E. (1987). The rise of family theory: A historical and critical analysis. In M. B. Sussman & S. K. Steinmetz (Eds.). *Handbook on marriage and the family* (pp. 81-103). NY: Plenum.

Index

Note: Page numbers followed by f indicate figures; page numbers followed by t indicate tables.

Ablon, J., 178
Achtenberg, R., 26
Adultery, in Lithuania, 75
Alanen, L., 109
All Our Kin, 6
Askham, J., 28

Backett, K.C., 28
Bahr, H.M., 94
Ball, D.W., 24,31
Bane, M., 175
Barrett, M., 27,110
Baudrillard, J., 62
Beavin, J.H., 192
Behavioral family therapy, 200
Bell, N.W., 94
Bender, D.R., 31
Bender, E., 174
Berg-Cross, L., 166
Berger, P.L., 7,28
Berke, D.L., 173
Bernard, J., 211,214
Bernardes, J., 21,61,67,68
Beutler, I., 175
Bhatia, S., 163
Bolstad, T., 101
Boss, P., 96,185
Broderick, C., 95-96
Brown, M.M., 216
Buck, N., 31
Burns, L.H., 127
Burr, W.R., 34-35,175,220

Caplan, G., 183
Caplow, T., 94
Caregiver(s)
    family, described, 150-153
    of infirm elderly, 153-155
Caregiving
    defined, 146
    defining families in terms of,
        155-156
    family, 149-156
Caregiving patterns
    defining families through, 145-159
    in family time periods, 147-149
Censorship, in defining family, 216
Chadwick, B.A., 94
Chapman, N., 178
Cheal, D., 21,30,61-62
Childlessness, 121-133
    as cause of men divorcing women,
        in Jewish tradition, 47
    in Sweden, 122-131
        couple and the social network,
            123-124
        home and the social network,
            125
        home ownership, 124-125
        involuntary childlessness and
            the social network, 125-126
        men and women's stories,
            differences between, 129-131
        men as husband-father, 128-129
        non-fathers, 126-127
        non-mothers, 126-127
        women and friends, 127-128
        women at work, 128